Advance Praise for *The Caregiving Wife's Handbook*

"This book is a must-read for women and men who are caring for their sick or disabled spouses. Many find themselves with a new 24/7, year-round job that leaves them feeling stressed, angry, lonely, guilty, and overwhelmed. Readers will find inspiration, understanding, and practical advice on how to make the best of this ultimate expression of marital love and devotion. Kudos to Diana Denholm for writing this important new resource for the spousal caregivers who are the unsung heroes of our time."

— James P. Firman, EdD
President and CEO, *National Council on Aging*

"Our AARP members tell us that one of the most difficult challenges they face is caring for a spouse or loved one who has become disabled or terminally ill. In *The Caregiving Wife's Handbook*, Dr. Dehnolm provides the tools and practical advice caregivers need to navigate these rough waters and to emerge at peace with themselves and their loved ones."

— A. Barry Rand
CEO, AARP

"Family caregivers have been told time and again to take care of themselves so they can be good caregivers. As Dr. Denholm responds, 'Don't they understand that we would if we could?' Finally there is a handbook that gives caregivers not only permission but also tools to identify feelings, stop feeling guilty, and learn how to communicate. This could well be the way to overcome the biggest barrier to getting respite, and ultimately the personal peace, needed to carry on in the caregiving role."

— Jill Kagan, MPH, Program Director
ARCH National Resp̶i̶t̶e̶ ̶N̶e̶t̶w̶o̶r̶k̶ ̶a̶n̶d̶ ̶R̶e̶s̶o̶u̶r̶c̶e̶ ̶C̶e̶n̶t̶e̶r̶

"Sharing her personal journey and drawing upon her knowledge of psychology, Dr. Denholm provides the tools that helped her and so many others.

"Understanding that everyone's path is different, her narrative is inclusive and easily adaptable for all. There is no judgment of personal circumstances, and we are offered guidance on mitigating conflict, expressing emotions, and moving forward.

"Although written from a wife's unique viewpoint I saw myself on most pages.

"This book will empower and enlighten you—you are not alone."
— Lawrence Bocchiere III
President, Well Spouse Association

"This book is long overdue. Based on her personal experience and many years as a psychotherapist, Dr. Denholm provides well-written, good, solid, and practical advice. Couples should read this handbook long before one of them becomes ill. Learning what she teaches will prevent much turmoil and distress at the time of a long-term or terminal illness. Although many circumstances are different, husbands taking care of wives also will benefit from her advice.

"Mental-health professionals, particularly marriage and family therapists, should read this book as it clarifies the responsibilities and rights of both the caregiver and the ill person.

"To my knowledge, nobody has given such sound advice to wives under these distressing circumstances nor helped teach wives to cope in the absence of genuine understanding from friends and society in general."
— Alejandro Villalobos, MD, Psychiatrist
Diplomate American Board of Psychiatry
Private Practice and Hospital Staff Psychiatrist Palm Beach and Michigan
Former Associate Professor of Psychiatry and
Former Director of Mental Health, Bogota, Colombia

The
CAREGIVING
WIFE'S
HANDBOOK

To John Stowell Sammond,
the elegant man who lived
the other side of my story.

To the six women who generously
shared themselves,
their stories, their wisdom,
and their friendship.

To the women and men
who are living their stories now.

Ordering
Trade bookstores in the U.S. and Canada please contact:

Publishers Group West
1700 Fourth Street, Berkeley CA 94710
Phone: (800) 788-3123   Fax: (800) 351-5073

Hunter House books are available at bulk discounts for textbook course
adoptions; to qualifying community, health-care, and government
organizations; and for special promotions and fund-raising.
For details please contact:

Special Sales Department
Hunter House Inc., PO Box 2914, Alameda CA 94501-0914
Phone: (510) 865-5282   Fax: (510) 865-4295
E-mail: ordering@hunterhouse.com

Individuals can order our books from most bookstores,
by calling (**800**) **266-5592**, or from our website at
www.hunterhouse.com

The
*C*AREGIVING
WIFE'S
HANDBOOK

Caring for Your Seriously Ill Husband,
Caring for Yourself

DIANA B. DENHOLM, PHD, LMHC

Hunter House
PUBLISHERS

For further information please contact:

Hunter House Inc., Publishers
PO Box 2914
Alameda CA 94501-0914

Library of Congress Cataloging-in-Publication Data
Denholm, Diana B.
The caregiving wife's handbook : caring for your seriously ill husband, caring for yourself / Diana B. Denholm.
p. cm.
Includes bibliographical references and index.
ISBN 978-0-89793-605-7 (pbk.)
1. Terminally ill—Psychology. 2. Terminal care—Psychological aspects.
3. Husbands—Death—Psychological aspects. 4. Wives—Psychology.
5. Women caregivers—Psychology. I. Title.
BF789.D4D47 2011
362.17'508655—dc23   2011023474

Project Credits
Cover Design: Brian Dittmar Graphics, Inc.   Interns: Erica M. Lee, Jack Duffy
Book Production: John McKercher   Acquisitions Assistant: Elizabeth Kracht
Developmental Editor: Kelsey Comes   Publicity & Marketing: Sean Harvey
Copy Editor: Heather Wilcox   Right Coordinator: Candace Groskreutz
Proofreader: John David Marion   Order Fulfillment: Washul Lakdhon
Indexer: Candace Hyatt   Administrator: Theresa Nelson
Managing Editor: Alexandra Mummery   Computer Support: Peter Eichelberger
Senior Marketing Associate: Reina Santana
Customer Service Manager: Christina Sverdrup
Publisher: Kiran S. Rana

Printed and bound by Bang Printing, Brainerd, Minnesota
Manufactured in the United States of America

9 8 7 6 5 4 3 2 1   First Edition   11 12 13 14 15

Contents

Important Note

The material in this book is intended to provide a review of information regarding managing mental-health issues for a wife whose husband is critically ill or dying. Every effort has been made to provide accurate and dependable information. The contents of this book have been compiled through professional research and in consultation with medical and mental-health professionals. However, professionals in these fields have differing opinions, and some of the information may become outdated.

Therefore, the publisher, authors, and editors, as well as the professionals quoted in the book cannot be held responsible for any error, omission, or dated material. The authors and publisher assume no responsibility for any outcome of applying the information in this book. If you have questions concerning the application of the information described in this book, consult a qualified medical, mental-health, legal, or finance professional.

Acknowledgments

A special thanks to Colleen Churm who did the critical read on the first version of the handbook and continued to lend support along its lengthy journey.

Thanks to the Hunter House professionals: Liz Kracht, acquisitions, who spotted the manuscript; Kiran Rana, publisher, who recognized its value; and Alex Mummery, managing editor, who edited with heart and engaged and guided the wonderful editorial staff through the book's development. Readers will benefit from the additional clarity each editor instilled.

Thank you to Dr. David Shern, CEO of Mental Health America, for being the first to recognize the merit of and to endorse the handbook. Thank you to Barry Rand, CEO of AARP; Dr. Jim Firman of the National Council on Aging; Larry Bocchiere, president of the Well Spouse Association; Jill Kagan of the National Respite Network; and my good friend and colleague Dr. Alejandro Villalobos for the very thoughtful and meaningful endorsements each person provided.

I've also appreciated the curiosity about the project and the support of my close friends who *knew* this project would come to fruition.

Introduction: What's Happening to My Life?

When a husband dies suddenly of a heart attack, stroke, or accident, it is tragic. But when a husband is in the process of dying for many months or for many years, the experience is quite different. Somehow, on top of dealing with that tragedy, a wife must figure out how to make a strange and foreign life work while everything around her is falling apart.

Whether due to illness or to a catastrophic injury, the challenges during this time are endless and extreme. Although sometimes wives can step back and look at the blessings and gifts their challenges bring, the reality is that going through this period with their husbands often isn't the beautiful, fulfilling, warm, spiritually uplifting, honored, or revered journey often portrayed. I know, because not only did I interview women who were caregivers, I was also the caregiver for my husband for 11½ years. Most women I interviewed felt as though they'd scream if they heard one more person tell them what a *gift* their situation was. The mere mention of that view made them feel guilty, because that was not what they were experiencing. And because they were not experiencing this set of circumstances as a "gift," for some, real life had become a dirty little secret.

Life changes dramatically, and with these changes come pressures, issues, questions, complaints, and problems. Although one might expect complaints of being fatigued or overwhelmed, many women are also steamed about a number of nonmedical issues relating to their husbands' dying. No two situations are alike, but I'm sure you've found that your life is changing radically and that you're facing situations you never dreamed existed. And you've likely found that although a lot of information and help is available for those "final days" and the grieving afterward, there are no written instructions for making life work during the long months and years you're facing as a caregiver.

In addition to being a caregiver, I am a board-certified medical psychotherapist. Even with my training and professional experience, like others in this caregiving situation, I found no direction for handling the myriad problems involved with my circumstances. So I know, firsthand, what you're facing. When we are with husbands who are dying, the day-to-day matters of our role in their care, our previous roles, our self-care, our ongoing lives, household management, sleep, sex and intimacy, changes in and strains on our marriages, and current and future finances are all right in our face. Practical issues continue that require action on our parts. Some require important communication between us and our husbands. Which issues should I discuss or shouldn't I discuss with my husband? How do I sort out these issues? And then, how should I handle the issues themselves?

I often heard myself say, "I'm learning far more than I ever cared to." What I learned ran the gamut from complex finances, to operating sprinkler-system pumps, to decoding insurance explanation-of-benefits reports, to getting blood out of white carpet, to dressing wounds, to changing a catheter bag—to name a few. For caregivers, every day brings new challenges and often-unwelcome changes to life. Life becomes an on-again, off-again affair that tosses us about in the process—the roller-coaster ride from hell. Though the gift of time allows us to prepare and say all the loving things we wish, it also provides a lot of time for severe stresses and problems to develop. This situation can debilitate caregivers, and it provides too many opportunities to say and do things we could regret.

Without specific direction, we can find ourselves at our wit's end. Sometimes the woman is married to the love of her life, and sometimes she isn't. Some marriages strengthen, while others disintegrate. Some women are in abusive relationships and find that the abuse continues, and even increases, during these times. Others find, much to their surprise, that *they* become emotionally and, sometimes, physically abusive to their husbands. Some find they start or increase alcohol and substance abuse (including food) to get through the years. Some have affairs for emotional sustenance. Not a pretty picture.

Although you cannot avoid the fact that your husband is going to die, you can avoid an ugly experience resulting in irreparable damage and regret and, instead, create a far different outcome. You and your husband can make it through these challenges, including the death itself, emotionally whole and with compassion for yourself and for each other.

My husband has passed on, but amid the grief is a sense of peace and completion about his passing—not because he's dead and the issues and concerns have stopped, but because of how I handled the issues and concerns while he was alive. To make our lives work, I created and used a variety of tools that allowed me to have absolutely no regrets at the time he died. I wouldn't have done a single thing differently—and I still feel the same way. This book provides the necessary help and direction for you to do the same. These are the tools to help you create a prettier picture.

We often feel alone in our circumstances, even though more than 30 million women are caregivers to an ill person. Advances in medical technology result in more and more individuals being kept alive longer. This longevity places more people in the stressful caregiving role, and for longer periods, than at any other time in history. Certainly some are taking care of parents, elderly relatives, close friends, or children. Although these situations share some similarities, major differences exist between caregiving for other types of people and caregiving for dying husbands. (I include in the term "husband" the person in a same-sex domestic life partnership who carries the typically masculine roles and duties.)

Some of the differences lie in the roles the dying people hold in our lives and the expectations we have for them. A husband's lengthy dying process is unique. Often we expect him to be with us our entire life or perhaps to be taken quickly when it is *his time*. But we also expect him to be there for us in a variety of capacities we don't expect of the others. He is our lover. He is our partner. He is our best friend. And specific jobs and responsibilities, whether they be financial, practical, or otherwise are his domain. Because of these expectations, living with a dying husband is distinctly difficult. And the more months and years the dying process takes, the more complex the problems become.

One ironic distinction is that most wives don't label themselves, and aren't labeled by others, as caregivers. People tending to the other groups are given and claim the label, because this isn't their usual role. But a wife tends to remain a "wife" in the eyes of the world, because caregiving is her *expected* role. Generally she isn't considered a "caregiver" or given credit for that role. She is just *doing what a wife is supposed to do*.

I am not ignoring the plight of the husband. That experience is well covered in other books. Considering that, however, I remember a comment from a widower who had the experience of being a caregiver for his cancer-stricken wife and then contracting and dying of cancer himself: He said it was much easier being the one *with* cancer.

My Story

When I was two, my father had a heart attack that he survived. My family adjusted life to accommodate his weaknesses. As I grew up, I remember thinking that at any moment, he would die. When I was a senior in high school, he hemorrhaged and collapsed in his office, surviving only because a hospital was located across the street. Subsequently he developed skin cancer. Eventually the cancer spread to his brain, resulting in his death ten years later. I experienced all this from the point of view of a daughter, but I also hold vivid memories of watching my mother trying to cope with all this drama and trauma off and on for about forty years. I knew what the experience of caring for a dying person was like from the perspective of a daughter, but I didn't really know what my mother went through…then.

As an adult, new challenges came my way. My husband, sixteen years my senior, was very athletic and robust. A month after proposing marriage, he was diagnosed with colon cancer, with only a 20 percent survival prospect. Following surgery and chemo for a year, he not only survived but, after five years, was deemed "cured." A year or so after the cancer, he developed congestive heart failure. During his deterioration, he was placed on transplant lists and, after his health declined severely for four more years, was fortunate to receive a heart transplant. Following the transplant, a variety of body systems began to fail due to antirejection medications. The system failures resulted in his needing dialysis for kidney failure, having severe osteoarthritis, frequent bouts of gout, chronic urinary tract infections, a poorly functioning colon, diverticulosis and diverticular bleeds, hernias, chronic eyelid infections, skin cancers, fluctuating blood pressure, depression, a sleep disorder, free-floating blood clots, a choking disorder, and Parkinson's disease. His low blood pressure and various medicines resulted in temporarily clouded thinking. During his final months, he could pursue normal activities a few hours some days, but the majority of his time was spent either sleeping, at doctor's appointments, or receiving dialysis. Heart failure, falls, bleeds, and other traumas resulted in many emergency room visits and ambulance rides. He also had severe hearing loss in both ears. Although he often was described as "the Energizer Bunny," basically he was dying for more than eleven and a half years. On 31 January 2006 he made his transition.

What You Can Expect from This Book

As Susan, whom you will meet in Chapter 1, says about living with her dying husband, "It's not glamorous. It's just hard work!" You will learn how to do this hard work. And, as you come to know the women in the book, you will no longer feel alone in your difficult challenges. You'll gain insight, knowledge, and wisdom from their candidly shared responses. This information will enable you to develop compassionate empowerment over your own life.

In *The Caregiving Wife's Handbook* you will learn:

🌱 how to handle the many difficult questions you'll have—and those you wouldn't even think to ask:

- Is it normal for me to think…?
- What do I do when…?
- How do I ask him about…?
- Do I really have to…?
- How can I…?
- What do I do when he won't discuss…?
- What do I say when they say…?

🌿 how to recognize the issues that bother you and decide which ones need to be discussed with your husband or shared with others

🌿 methods for raising difficult topics with your husband and how to create Understandings between the two of you

🌿 the fine-line issues you'll have to walk and how to walk them

🌿 which problems you can expect and solutions for them

🌿 what Cathy, Fran, Tina, Jean, Susan, Mary, and I thought and experienced, and our survival tips

🌿 roles you should take and those you should avoid

🌿 what is "normal" in what you're experiencing and feeling

🌿 to take care of yourself so you can survive and even have fun

🌿 specific do's and don'ts to make your life simpler

🌿 how to manage your balancing act with greater ease

Allow this book to support you through your entire journey—all the way through *your* husband's final days.

chapter *1*

Examining Our Issues

I'M SURE MANY ISSUES are surfacing both about your husband
and between you and your husband. And, just as elsewhere in
life, usually each issue has two sides. Unlike other times when
you might have championed your side, you probably aren't now,
because your husband is dying. Even when it is something really
important, you decide just to let it go and not make a fuss so his
life is more pleasant. The fact that your husband is dying tends
to encourage you to lean toward his interests and needs. Knowing the situation is temporary, you give yourself permission to
tip even farther to his side. After all, this situation won't last forever.... Allowing yourself to lean in his direction seems fine for
awhile, but over the months and years of his illness, sometimes
you seem so far off balance that it takes every ounce of energy to
keep from falling. That is unhealthy for everyone.

As you look at the practical issues, emotional issues, and social and familial issues that the following chapters discuss, you'll
notice they are not about one person being right and the other

being wrong. Rather, the interests, needs, and requirements of you and your husband may just be different, or even opposite.

Fortunately, rather than losing your balance completely or continuously fighting when you reach an impasse, you can have special discussions to clarify and to settle issues, creating what I call "Understandings." *These Understandings are what will make life work.* Rather than ignoring or going around issues, Understandings allow us to put our relationships in the best balance possible and to make life work for us and for our husbands.

Even in households with the best communication, some issues are daunting to raise. Because some of our concerns may be based in fear, it can be very difficult to express them. But leaving some issues buried may lead to extra burdens after our husbands pass. Not discussing other issues definitely results in increased stress and growing resentment toward our husbands, ourselves, and others. Unfortunately, those stresses and resentments may lead to a diminished quality of life for both, emotional and physical exhaustion and illness for us, and even emotional and physical abuse of our husbands by us!

Reluctance to have discussions may come from our past experiences with difficult issues or from trying to discuss *anything* with our husbands. Other issues are just so new or uncomfortable, we have no clue about how to raise them. Some may seem so unlikely to be resolved that talking about them doesn't seem worth the effort.

You may wish to talk about certain issues, and your husband doesn't, or won't. This situation is very common, because many people, especially men, don't like to talk about topics involving their feelings, matters they deem to be their sole domain, or matters where they might have been failures. Most likely, the topics you need to discuss now are reminders and reinforcement of your husband's deterioration and his looming demise. For your husband, avoiding these discussions may be like refusing to make a will with the hope of fooling death.

It may be that he wants to talk but you don't. This occurrence is also common, because many women don't want to face the fact that their husbands are dying. Even when they're told their husbands are terminally ill, understandably, they try to stay in hopeful denial and are afraid to leave that safe place. Wives also realize they'll have to deal with unfamiliar things, whether they are the finances, the furnace, or the funeral arrangements. It is important to know that all these reactions and responses are not only normal but expected.

Any conversation about these difficult topics takes thoughtful preparation. The more difficult the topic, the more thoughtful the preparation. The tools I give you may make it seem as though you'll be conducting business, and that's pretty accurate. This is some of the most important business of your life, and you want to have things go as well as possible. Without preparation, you may end up with the opposite of the result you want.

If your husband is a businessman, he may find this somewhat businesslike approach more appealing and less threatening, because you're speaking his language. And, fortunately, what you may find is that your husband is extremely relieved that you are raising these concerns, particularly if he didn't know how to talk to *you* about them. He may have been trying to protect you from unpleasantness, and now he doesn't have to. Even though you may think your husband doesn't know he's dying, it may honestly surprise you to know that it is most likely no secret to him!

Your preparation comes in several parts that are discussed in this and the next three chapters. **First,** included in this chapter, is answering some questions for yourself. In Chapter 2, the **second** step is explained, which is choosing your topics. Chapter 3 presents the **third** step, which is becoming familiar with simple communication tools. It is very important to complete this step *before* attempting the next step. The remaining steps are included in Chapter 4. The **fourth** is making a date or appointment for a discussion with your husband and determining the best possible physical environment for that date. The **fifth** is preparing yourself emotionally just before your date to encourage mutual respect, compassion, and kindness to come forth. The **sixth** is having your date and creating Understandings.

Using these tools will make your experience much easier. However, you won't be perfect. Even though I created many of the techniques and have used them myself for many years, I don't always do them correctly—and that's okay. This is not about perfection. We are human and we won't be perfect.

Prompts to Start Planning

Below are twenty-four prompts (cues, suggestions, ideas) to think about. At this point, it is good just to have a brainstorming session and to write down your responses. Nothing that affects you is off-limits for your list. The issues don't have to be related to health or dying. Because marriage goes on, you may want to talk about ordinary issues too. Whether it is a toilet seat that stays up, disrespectful behavior, the annoying in-laws who stick their noses into your business, or crumbs in the bed: If it bothers you, it should be put on your list. You should include as many items as you like. Feel free to add to the list at any time. If you think of something I didn't, add your own categories. If you are having difficulty starting, you might want to look ahead to the responses given by the six women who shared their lists of concerns, which may give you a jump start.

I begin with prompts about anger, because these are probably the easiest to answer. Many of your emotions—whether fear, pain, depression, anxiety, or feeling overwhelmed—are more than likely going to surface as anger at this time, so this is a good subject to start with. Most of the women I speak with are quite angry about several aspects of life with their dying husbands. Of course, most outsiders don't know that, because the women tend to put on happy faces. Also, they're afraid of sounding like heartless shrews because of their complaints. After all, to much of the outside world, they are only suffering *inconvenience* while their husbands are facing death.

Prompts to Help You Sort Out Your Concerns

1. I am angry about the following things…
2. I am frustrated about or with…
3. What really annoys me is…
4. What I hate the most is…
5. I'm angry with myself about…
6. I'm afraid that…
7. I'm afraid of…
8. I need to know…
9. I feel guilty about…
10. I want to do these things for my husband…
11. I don't want to do these things for my husband…
12. I don't think I can…
13. I want him to…
14. I don't want him to…
15. What am I supposed to do about…
16. What do I do when…
17. Why does he…
18. Why doesn't he…
19. What do I say to people about…
20. What concerns me a lot is…
21. I don't know how to…
22. I don't expect anything to be done about this, but I want you to know…
23. This is something I need to say to you…
24. And something else I really want to say is…

Responses from the Group

Each of the six wives responded to the twenty-four prompts. Although they shared many more responses, below I've included just one response to each prompt from each wife. All the names are fictitious, but the responses of Cathy, Fran, Tina, Jean, Susan, and Mary are real or slightly modified versions of what they said. Some of my own responses are mixed in with theirs. These are shared not only to help you start thinking but to give you some idea of the range of normal reactions. No judgment is placed on any of these responses. As I've taught my clients over the past thirty-five years:

🙢 *Emotions are neither good nor bad; they just are.*

— Cathy —

Cathy is a waitress who was married for forty-six years. She and her husband, Craig, have three children and several grandchildren. Even though Craig was the love of her life, he was a verbally abusive husband. As they both approached seventy, Craig developed colorectal cancer complicated by overradiation and overmedication. He was severely diabetic and had a bad reaction to insulin, which caused him to have a stroke. Craig had been terminally ill for six years while Cathy was the primary breadwinner and caregiver. Craig passed away while this book was being written. Shortly after his passing, Cathy suffered a heart attack and has had an uphill battle recovering from that. She shared the following thoughts while Craig was still alive:

> I'm so angry when others offer to help him, and he pretends he's so strong and doesn't need their help. Of course when they leave, he expects me to wait on him hand and foot while he screams at me. It's so frustrating, because even though he's coherent and sharp and pretty strong physically, he expects me to wait on him like I'm his servant —

even though I'm the sole support of the family and work long, hard hours. He manages to go to the baseball field and chat with his buddies but somehow manages to not be able to do anything for himself at home. But what *really* annoys the hell out of me is that he doesn't want to have sex. Yet he acts like the lack of sex only affects *him*. He's so selfish! But what I hate most is that when I'm trying to fix him a meal, he gets in my way. Then something falls and spills or breaks, and he has a fit and threatens to pack a bag and move out. Here I am, trying to help. He doesn't appreciate it, and he makes it worse. Sometimes I wish he *would* move out! But I'm really angry at myself for not standing up to him more. I let him walk all over me. Even though he yells at me, I'm afraid that if I don't monitor his eating, he will kill himself with what he eats. He's diabetic and eats horribly. You'd think he'd know better.

And I'm so afraid I won't have money to live on after he dies. I don't know what money there is, and I'm afraid to ask him, because he gets angry when I bring it up. I really need to know what money is there for me after he goes. He doesn't bring up the finances, and I'm afraid to. I don't know anything about money, except that I'm the one who has to earn it!

But, you know, I do feel guilty about being angry with him and talking back to him. Sometimes I really let him have it. I guess we communicate by yelling and screaming at each other. Yet I love him so much that I want to be the one he cries with. I want to be that person who is there for him. He won't share the tears, but I'm the one he takes his anger out on, particularly in public, and I don't want to be his punching bag.

His mood swings are so horrible; I don't think I can keep going with life being like a seesaw. I'm never sure how he'll react to me from one day to the next. I'm frightened and tired, and I want him to stop screaming at me! But even when I'm really pissed off at him, I really don't want him to die.

Gee, what the hell am I supposed to do about the smell? His bedroom has such a smell—it makes me sick to go in to help him. Yes, he's got a colostomy bag, but he has the strength to get up and take care of that himself. He's just content to live in that hellhole. I don't know what to do when he doesn't care for himself the way he should, and his room is so smelly I can't stand to go in. But somebody's got to take care of him.

You know, I don't understand why he always acts like my ideas are no good and then does the very same thing when someone else suggests it. Why doesn't he treat me nicer? Doesn't he know I am working hard to make a living and take care of him—and that this is really hard on me, too? And when people ask me how he's doing, I don't know what to say to them. I don't want to talk about it at all, but I don't want to be rude.

What really concerns me a lot is that I don't know what I'll live on after he dies. I'd really like to tell him that he's selfish, even with our daughter, but I don't dare.

I know he can't do anything about it now, but I'd really like to tell him I don't think it's fair that he's squandered the money we needed to live on. He always had some "deal" or some "scheme" that was supposed to make us rich, and here we are—about as far from that as you can get.

When I'm not angry, I'd really like to tell him that I always think of him the way he was before. I know his mind isn't the same. I know he's really not trying to be mean to me. And I guess I'd really like to tell him that it would have been nice if he had made things easier for me, been nicer, and helped with my future rather than just being concerned about himself and his "deals," but I know that probably wouldn't accomplish anything.

⎯ Fran ⎯

Fran, a school teacher in her fifties, had been married to Frank for twenty years. A second marriage for both, she has three grown children. Frank was dying of emphysema and had been a very ardent smoker. Because his brain was deprived of oxygen, often his mental state was a bit confused. Fran continued to juggle work and home. From time to time, one of the children visited and offered some help. One lived nearby and was able to give Fran breaks as well as be an understanding confidant. Fran shared these comments during Frank's illness:

> You know what really frosts me is that he *caused* this with his smoking. Even though he had many early warnings that the cigarettes were damaging his lungs, he just kept right on. Now *I* have to deal with the results. And I think he is still sneaking cigarettes! And who knows how much damage he's caused to my health over the years?
>
> Here's something that really frustrates me. All of our phones are portable. Frank answers the phone in one room, then calls to me to ask a question. Even though he's still able to bring the phone to where I am, he expects *me* to stop what I'm doing, get up, and go to him. He may be sick, but I'm sick and tired of that! Another really annoying thing is talking to people who presume to know what I'm going through. One person said he knew exactly what I was going through, because his parents were ill for several years and it was so hard when he went to see them *once a year!* Like that's really the same thing!
>
> I really hate it when he turns down help from other people and gets himself into physical trouble. He'll try to fix something himself but gets so exhausted that he can't finish and has to go to bed. Then along with everything else I'm taking care of, I get stuck taking more care of him *plus* fixing whatever it was he tried to fix!

It may not make sense to say it, but when I fight with myself to take care of me, I get angry with myself. I should be able to know it's okay to take care of myself and should just be doing it! And I'm afraid he'll go on living forever like this and I'll *never* be free. And I'll totally lose who I am. I'm also afraid of him having a painful death. As much as he annoys me and makes me angry, I'd really hate to have him go through that—and I pray his death will be peaceful. But I really need to know when he'll die. Each day is like waiting for the other shoe to drop. I can't make plans for him, and I can't make plans for me. I can't keep stopping everything for his final days, because he recovers a bit, then gets worse, then recovers a bit—so who knows when the end will come? And, yes, I do feel guilty about wanting this to be over. But how much more can I take?!

Until the very end, I want to be there for him emotionally so this is easier for him. But I don't want to be his scrub nurse! I trained to be a teacher, not a scrub nurse. Even if I knew how, that's not the role I want to have with him. And I don't think I can handle him physically anymore, anyway. He's too heavy, and he's too unsteady. Instead of relying on me all the time because it's easier and nicer for him, I want him to use more outside help that's available. There are other people who can do things for him…if he'd just stop turning them down!

I don't want him to suffer now or at the end. But what am I supposed to do about it if he won't follow doctor's orders or use information the doctor has given him? He's just setting himself up for trouble, and for suffering because of the trouble he creates. And I don't know what to do when he refuses to wear his Depends and he messes up the bed. I know he's embarrassed by the thought of wearing Depends, but you'd think he'd be more embarrassed waking up with the bed full of poop! Why does he have to act so stubborn when he knows the things I suggest are helping him? Why does he still refuse to do most of it? Why doesn't he just do these things so he can relax and enjoy his last days?

A lot of my friends at work ask about how he's doing. What do I say to people about what really goes on here? There's so much I'd be mortified about if anyone knew. I just can't answer them. And what concerns me a lot is that something will happen to him and I won't know what to do about it. What if he gets confused and wanders out for a walk and falls? I'm really good as a teacher, but, like I said before, I'm not trained as a nurse. I'm just not good at this at all.... And I don't know how to deal with his mental confusion. I'm not sure when he hears me and understands me, or not. He sort of acts like he's listening but gets upset if I ask if he heard and understood what I told him. I don't know how bad the lack of oxygen has made things—will he even remember what I said?

Even though nothing can be done about this, I want him to know that it just breaks my heart that he could have prevented all of this. I need to say to him that I'm truly sorry he's going through this. Even though I complain about the impact this has had on my life, I'm still really sorry that he is dying from this.

And when I've really had it up to here, I want to say to him that I feel like you've stolen my years with your illness and that you couldn't care less that you did!

— Tina —

Tina has been married for forty-five years, and Tom is the only husband still alive at the time of this writing. Tom has grown children from a previous marriage. Tina is about 5'5" and slender, and Tom is about 6'5" and full-bodied. She was a high-powered professional woman prior to her marriage. Tom suffers from severe alcoholism, dementia, and heart problems. He has been seriously ill for twelve years and has almost died several times from the interplay of alcohol, heart problems, and severe falls. The combination of alcoholism and dementia results in impaired judgment, which puts him at constant physical risk of death from falls, severe burns, or mistakes related to self-medication. Tina is now in her early eighties, and Tom in his mid-eighties. Tina offered these responses:

I am *muy enfadado* [very angry] about him sneaking booze. I give him Antabuse to keep him from drinking. But when I am out of the house, he invites his friends over and talks them into sneaking some liquor in for him. Then *I* have to deal with him when he gets sick from it.

I'm frustrated about the way he takes showers. He just goes in, gets wet, and comes out. He doesn't clean himself. I have to send someone in to clean him or do it myself. He still could do this, but he just doesn't bother. He's like a little kid who goes through the motions, because he really doesn't understand the purpose of the shower. Of course, then I have to have that smell around if he "misses" while cleaning.

What really annoys me is when other people try to interfere with what I feel is necessary. Like with the Antabuse—they think it's mean. They don't know. They don't live with him! They don't know what he's like when he's drunk. He's a danger to himself and to me! And what I hate the most is the fact that he did this to himself! He's had lots of chances to get off the booze with professional help, but he always messes it up.

Well, I'm not angry with myself about anything, nor do I feel guilty about anything. I'm doing the best for him I can and am treating him very well. I like the way I'm doing things and wouldn't change any of it! I'm not afraid of anything, but I'm afraid that he will fall again. He's fallen so many times. I can't pick him up, and he keeps getting injured. He's got cuts and bruises all over him.

I need to know what he's up to when I'm not around. He's gotten himself into some big problems I'm too embarrassed to tell you about. All because of that damned drinking! Right now, all I want to do for him is cook and keep a nice house for him. I think he likes that I do those things for him. But I don't want to be our source of income or his nurse. He has plenty of money, and I don't want him squandering that so he has to dip into mine.

I really don't think I can put up with some of his sneaky behavior. It's caused us so many problems already, and I feel like I'll walk into some bad surprise every time I return to the house. I just want him to behave. How hard is that? I don't want him to sneak alcohol and make himself worse. He's got enough problems without adding that to them.

What am I supposed to do about things he refuses to discuss? I think it's getting time for us to move to assisted living, but he won't discuss selling the house. [Eventually they moved to assisted living.] He gets so angry if I even start to mention it. He's so big and scary. Nobody ever sees that side of him but me. He's always so polite if others are around. I feel like I need to keep people around all the time just so he'll be nice!

What do I do when people criticize me for taking care of myself? They think I'm a bad wife, because I go out to lunch with friends or go to see my family. I have to get away once in awhile, and some people are really mean to me when I tell them about it. A few have stopped being friends with me.

Why does he keep putting himself in harm's way by doing all that drinking? Why doesn't he just take his medicine so he feels better? He seems to be happier when he uses the medicine and doesn't drink. It doesn't make any sense to me. So what do I say to people about what's really wrong with him? I don't want them to know that besides the dementia, he drinks and gets into some big problems by acting foolish. But they keep asking. What do I say to people?

What concerns me is how I'll find people who are willing to work with him—people I can trust. Some people aren't willing to work with him because he's so big. It's too hard for them. And we've had other people who have sneaked booze to him and taken our money. It's just awful.

I don't think there's anything I don't know how to do, so I'll have to say *nada* to that. Even though I don't expect anything to be done about it, I want him to know that I really miss my healthy, sober Tom. That was the person I fell in love with, and I'd like him back. I need to say to him that I really appreciate that every day he tells me how lucky he is that he has me. It seems that in spite of the dementia and drinking, there still is a part of him that knows and appreciates all that I do. It makes me cry when he says that to me.

On the other hand, something I'd really like to say is, "What's the matter with you? Why don't you stop killing yourself and ruining both of our lives? You're making matters worse than they need to be, and I'm sick and tired of it!"

— Susan —

Susan is a homemaker who was married to Sam for twenty-five years. They have grown children from his previous marriage. She and Sam were in their late fifties. He had Merkel cell carcinoma for six years. It was considered incurable but treatable. Sam seemed to have severe psychological problems as well. He'd go through serious declines and short remissions, followed by more serious declines. He was considered terminal for four of the last six years of his illness. Susan shared the following while he was alive:

I am angry about him not including me in it, in his illness. Even though I go to doctor's appointments with him, he won't let me participate. Because he chooses to do everything his way without my input, I feel he has cut me out of the final act of this marriage. He doesn't share his thoughts about the way he is feeling. He's very withdrawn and introverted. It seems that not only is he dying, the marriage is dying along with him.

He always acts like his health issues are worse than everyone's. I have a cold, so he thinks he has pneumonia. Yes, he's got a terminal illness, but it's so frustrating when he does this about anything and everything. Then what really annoys me is that he uses his illness as a license to be beastly. He is just so awful to me, even though I really have tried to make things nice for him. Sam won't take care of himself and expects me to feel sorry for him, and that really annoys the hell out of me. He was supposed to get twenty-four-hour urine samples every month to monitor when he was and wasn't in remission. When the carcinoma is active, that shows up in the tests, and he can be treated. Well, he lets months go by without the testing. Recently he had the test showing the carcinoma is very active, and he could have prevented that or at least started treatment sooner. I just hate that, because it doesn't need to be that way, and it affects both of us.

I'm angry with myself for not being able to be nicer to him and his relatives. But they just cause so many problems every time they visit, it turns me upside down. I'm afraid that when he's forgetful and doesn't make sense, he might do something dangerous or with serious consequences. He's just so unpredictable, and I never know what he's up to. And I'm afraid of the silence in the house and that we are developing bad patterns and habits rather than facing our problems.

It's just easier to be quiet, but I know that's not a good thing for us.

I need to know that people care about me too. Everybody asks about Sam, but they never ask how I'm doing. Don't they notice? Don't they care?

I feel guilty about getting so angry with Sam. I start out thinking I'll say something in a nice way, but then I lose it. It's not good this way. And what I really want to do for him is to be his lover, but he won't let me. Instead, I'm his verbal punching bag, and I certainly don't want to be that for him! I really don't think I can do this much longer. I still want him to be my lover, but he won't let that happen. He doesn't want sex anymore, but he's certainly able to do it. I don't want him to shut me out of his life, but that's what he's done.

What am I supposed to do about having his visitors at the house who make everything worse? I know they are his family members, and he has a right to have them visit. Everything is pretty awful while they are here and interfering, and things get even worse after they leave. Talk about being between a rock and a hard place! What do I do when people think we don't like them because we turn down invitations? They don't know he's so sick. He doesn't want them to know. Instead, they just drop us socially, even though getting out probably would do wonders for us both.

Why does he just barge through things, not caring, acting like a slob when he could do otherwise? He used to be so careful about his appearance and was a real gentlemen. What do I say to people about the fact that we don't socialize because he won't change his clothes or get clean anymore? I feel like I'm living with Howard Hughes! He acts and looks that bad! Why doesn't he try harder to get better? He could be better, if he just chose to do so. I never know what's going on in his head, and that's what concerns me a lot. It's exhausting mentally having all the responsibilities. I have to be Mom, wife, secretary, bookkeeper. It would be easier if I could bounce ideas off him. He's a very bright man, and he used to let me bounce ideas off him, but he won't let me anymore.

You know, I just don't know anymore how to tell him things without getting angry. I wouldn't expect anything to be done if I told him this, but I'd like to tell him that I'm really pissed that he's dying! I really need to say, "Be my husband! Let me in! I'm suffering more by you keeping me out. It's as if you've already died for me." And furthermore, something else I'd really want to say is, "You're dying — I'm not! Just how long *is* terminal!?"

— Jean —

Jean was married for thirty-six years to the love of her life. Her husband, Joe, died of Parkinson's disease after a fifteen-year battle. Because they owned a business, Jean was used to working with her husband and sharing work and household responsibilities. She became the sole source of financial support during his dying process and became totally responsible for both the business and the home. Joe began getting sick in his mid-to-late forties, which was a big blow to them in the primes of their lives. Even though the death happened some years ago, all the emotions remain fresh for Jean, and she shares them below. She has created a wonderful life for herself since his passing. Thinking back, she shares thoughts from the time of his illness:

> I'm angry that I don't have a life anymore. Besides working, my husband and I took wonderful trips, went to concerts, went out dancing. Because he is dying, now that life is gone.
>
> I'm frustrated because he just won't move very fast. I know he can't, but it's still frustrating. I've got all these ex-tra things to do, and he gets in my way and slows me down. I could get so much more done if he weren't in my way all the time.
>
> But what really annoys me is that he had a neck injury that may have contributed to the Parkinson's. If he hadn't been so stubborn and done something that hurt him, we probably wouldn't have this problem! I don't know how

many times I told him to be careful on the ladder. But he just wouldn't listen—and here we are now!

What I really hate is that damned whistle I gave him. I know it's hard for him to speak very loudly, so he needs it. But can't he let me just stay put ten minutes without the whistle? Sometimes I'd like to put it where the sun doesn't shine! One night he wet the bed three times, and I had a screaming fit. I had to change the sheets three times, on top of everything else I had to do that day. I'm really angry with myself for screaming at him—he couldn't help it.

I'm afraid that I just can't do it all. There is so much for me to do everywhere—work and home. I'm afraid of my dying as a result of taking care of him. Even with some help, I'm getting so worn out that I'm getting sick. I'm losing so much weight, and my doctor is really worried about me. Now that I have all this extra work, I need to know how to do the things he used to do. He was so handy around the house and fixed everything. I don't have the money to hire a handyman, so now it's up to me to learn these things—not that I have the energy for it.

I really want to be away from him. He's going through so much, but I just have to get away, or I'll get sick. I feel guilty about that. I do want to cook and clean the house. I think those are nice things for me to do. And I still want to be his best friend. But I don't want to be responsible for all the money and the care, too. These are not the things I want to do for my husband. As it is, I don't think I can do it all the way I think I should. I like to do things the right way.

I want him to get well. I don't want him to die. But what am I supposed to do about having enough energy to stay alive and take care of him? What can I do when I don't know how to fix something and don't have the money to pay someone to do it? Why does he have to be sick? He doesn't deserve this. Why doesn't he let go so he doesn't have to suffer anymore?

What do I say to people about how he's doing, particularly when they never ask how *I'm* doing? I just don't understand that. Do they think I'm a robot? How will I be able to get him in and out of his wheelchair and into and out of bed without hurting him or me? That's what concerns me a lot. I know this sounds silly, but I don't know how to fix the water heater. I'll have to wheel him over to it and have him walk me through the steps. He was so good at fixing anything!

Even though I don't expect anything to be done about this, I'd like to say to him that he doesn't deserve to suffer like this. He's a good man. And I also need to say that sometimes I think I will die of exhaustion. But I know that if I give up and die, there would be no one to take care of him.

Something else I'd really want to say to him is, "You ruined our retirement plans. We had to scrap them, and I missed my chance."

— Mary —

Mary and her husband, Mark, were retired. This second marriage for both began thirty years ago. Both had children and grandchildren from their previous marriages. Mark was dying of Parkinson's disease, which was diagnosed seven years prior to his death. Because both were in their seventies at the time of his illness, the normal effects of aging complicated their ability to deal with the unexpected changes. Perhaps because of his age, Mark's decline from Parkinson's seemed to be quite rapid. Money was not an issue, so they had greater options for care. He passed away in 2009. While he was alive, Mary shared:

I'm so angry, because he keeps asking me the same questions over and over and over, again and again and again. "Where are we going today?" "What am I doing today?" "What time are we going out?" "What are we having for dinner?" even though I've told him each thing several times. He just doesn't remember *anything* I tell him.

He doesn't shave. I'm embarrassed when we go out, because that always makes him look messy. His clothing is nice, because I pick that out for him. I am so frustrated by this, because we have the same situation day after day after day! But what really annoys me is that every time I ask about finances, he just says, "Ask my attorney." I feel guilty doing that, and I don't like feeling that way. Even though he tells me to do it, I feel like I'm going behind his back if I do. I want *him* to discuss it with me. *He* is my husband, not the attorney! These were supposed to be our relaxed and comfortable years, and he has ruined that for us. Even though he couldn't help it, it's messed up my life, and I hate him for that. I know that sounds awful, but I do.

I get embarrassed when he falls in public, but I know he can't help it. I'm angry with myself for feeling that way, but I can't help it. It really is embarrassing. It seems that all the decisions are on me, and I'm afraid that I won't be able to make important decisions for him, like where we will live or if he will want to keep living at home. And I'm afraid of not knowing about our money. How can I make decisions about anything if I don't know the finances? I really need to know about our finances.

I feel guilty that I don't want to wait on him. He expects it, and I am able to, but I just don't *want* to. I want to be his mate, but I don't want to be his servant. I've never had to deal with something like this before. And I don't think I can handle social things. Can I go out to dinner with people without him? Is that done? What would people think?

I want him to take better care of himself while he can. There are a lot of things he can do for himself that he isn't doing. I don't want him to embarrass himself because he becomes unkempt. And what am I supposed to do about having a normal life? How do I make that happen? What do I do when he won't talk about where we should live? Why does he act like I should drop my life to take care of him? I still want to enjoy life. Why doesn't he ask others to help him, not just me? There are a lot of people who can help, and we have the means to hire them.

What do I say to people about why he falls? They think he's drunk and just give me a look. He doesn't drink at all. Should I tell them he has Parkinson's or just smile and say nothing? And if I'm not the first person at his side to help, people think I don't care.

What concerns me a lot is how I can schedule things I need to do around his needs. I want to be a good wife, but I am getting older and don't want to give up what's left of my life. I just don't know how to handle a social life with a dying husband. Being active in society has always been of part of who we were and who I am. How can I make that still happen? I don't expect anything to be done about this, but I want him to know I don't always do things right away, because I feel like I'm in shock about what is happening. It's not that I don't care—I'm really in shock. That's why when he falls, I'm not always the first one at his side. I'm just so shocked to see it happen that I can't move. And I really need to say to Mark, "I'm so frightened about all of this that I'm never sure what to say to you."

And one more thing I'd really like to say is, "I just didn't expect to have to deal with this for the remaining years of my life. Yes, I thought you might die before I did, but I wasn't prepared to have this go on for years and years."

Processing Your Responses

You probably noticed some common themes among the statements made by these six women: money, intimacy, cleanliness, lack of concern for the wife, being a servant, etc. I'm guessing that many of the responses you just read are not all that differ-ent from your own. If you haven't done so yet, respond to the prompts yourself, remembering that nothing is off-limits. You may have as many answers as you wish for each prompt, and you may add even more later. One benefit of answering the prompts is it allows you to get some of these emotions and reactions out of your system. You'll be better off writing down the things you've been ashamed of thinking and feeling. By doing that, you'll take a big step to help balance your emotions. It takes en-ergy to hide those thoughts and feelings inside, and you don't have any to waste.

Now that you've identified major issues, you can begin pre-paring for the next steps to make life work—for you and for your marriage.

chapter 2

Organizing Answers and Choosing Discussion Topics

To make it easier to get started, sort your answers into four categories:

A. things I want to say but don't expect a response to

B. things I want to say but won't, because it won't make a difference

C. things I want to say but should only share with a friend

D. things I really need to talk about, know about, have resolved, or make a decision about

If you look at these categories, you'll see you have a safe place to put the really volatile or uncomfortable responses to the twenty-four prompts. And everyone has some of those types of responses! Now that you've seen what you'll do with them, you may want to go back and add more responses.

When your answers are complete, start by putting each one into one of the four categories. If you want, take four pieces of paper and write a category at the top of each. Then cut each answer into a strip and place it on the appropriate sheet of paper. Or, use a box for each category. This way it will be easy to go back and move the strips with your responses to different categories. Of course, this can all be done on a computer; there are many easy ways to do this sorting. Whatever method you choose, the sorting process is a great help, so you really need to do it.

Obviously, all the likely discussion topics end up in category D. Categories A and B are not wasted, however, because even just writing responses down in these categories helps you get some emotions out of your system. Your responses also clarify and help make sense of what has been bothering you. Sometimes you feel a general malaise and don't understand why until you write down these things. Those items can also be put in category C, if you choose to share with a friend or other confidant. You likely know which will be the hot items. For each item in your D category, double-check to make sure it doesn't belong in categories A, B, or C. Once you've started having discussions with your husband, using your new skills, you may want to move more items from category B to category C, because doing so could make a difference.

Even if you've finished your lists, do *not* bring up any topic with your husband at this time. It is important to learn how to set up a "date" or "appointment" for a discussion and to learn a few simple communication tools before starting this process. Everyone has a natural tendency to let loose with this information once the lists are made, but don't do it.

As you proceed, remember to keep in mind the concepts of mutual respect, compassion, and kindness, and that "mutual" means it works in both directions—toward you, too! You should include respect, compassion, and kindness toward yourself as you consider which items to put on the discussion table. Let's look a little more closely at the four categories.

Category A: Things I Want to Say but Don't Expect a Response To

Sometimes we just have to say what's on our mind. It can be something tender and caring, it can be a neutral piece of information, or it can be something very negative. What we put on the A list is up to us. I am reminded of a friend's daughter whose husband wasn't happy with his job, so he just went ahead and quit, without consulting her and without having a new position lined up. They had a young child at home, so his quitting created a strain in many ways. She was extremely upset, so she took him aside and said, "I have some things to say to you that I have to get off my chest. I'm only going to say them to you once, but I want you just to listen so I can get this out—and I don't want you to say anything back." She unloaded her anger and tears, and then it was done and never discussed again. I don't recommend her exact approach, because she prohibited him from responding, but what she did was healthier than letting her anger fester. And their relationship was strong enough for this technique to work.

Now let's see what the six wives chose for category A. Cathy chose, "I always think of you as the way you were before, and I know your mind isn't the same. I know you're not trying to be mean to me." Fran selected, "I'm truly sorry you're going through this." Tina, in a grateful mood, decided to put, "I really appreciate that every day you tell me how lucky you are that you have me."

Jean decided to share her frustration, fatigue, and fear when she picked, "Sometimes I think I will die of exhaustion. But I know that if I give up and die, there will be no one to take care of you." Susan was obviously impassioned when she chose to share, "Be my husband! Let me in! I'm suffering more by you keeping me out. It's as if you've already died for me, and I still want to be a part of your life. This is what marriage is about, when people stay and they haul each other to the doctor when they'd rather just run away. This is worse than living alone, because I have to face you shutting me out every day." Mary shared a common fear of doing something wrong and decided to say to her husband, "I'm so frightened about all of this that I'm never sure what to say to you."

Category B: Things I Want to Say but Won't, Because It Won't Make a Difference

You've probably heard the Einstein adage that doing the same thing over and over and expecting a different outcome is insanity. We've all done it. We repeatedly ask our husbands to put down the toilet seat, to stop leaving their socks on the floor, to remember to do this and that. Yet it never works.

But we need to consider that at this point in their decline it may not be possible for our husbands to comply. For instance, we may be annoyed that our husbands don't pick up their clothes, but perhaps they can't bend over or they get dizzy if they try. Or we may be annoyed because they forget to take certain pills at a specific time. However, they may be disoriented and not know which pills they are supposed to take or what time it is.

In looking at your list, you may see that some items just aren't that important in the whole scheme of things. Although something may be the "last straw" because other issues are raging, if those other issues improved, that "last straw" may not matter at all. Although it is not insanity, it is certainly a waste of time and energy to repeat the same behavior over and over again expecting a different outcome. However, it doesn't change the fact that you're angry about something and want to say so! Getting it out of your system, whether on paper or to a friend, is a healthy way to do that without inflicting emotional damage on another person or, ultimately, yourself.

Let's take a look at the responses the six wives chose for category B. Cathy knew she nagged Craig about many things that aggravated her. She chose, "You're strong enough to carry bats to the baseball field, but you won't lift a finger at home! Why don't you ever ask how I am? Why do you expect me to stand there and listen to you scream at me? I'm not your punching bag. I'd like you to clean up the bedroom so there's room for me in the bed. If you controlled your diet better, you wouldn't have as many problems with the diabetes. I know you're sneaking too much sugar and bad food."

You can feel Fran's anger and frustration as she shared, "It's bad enough that I have to do extra work because you can't do any. But now there are extra duties in taking care of you, and you make messes you don't have to. So now it seems like I have four times the work I had before! It isn't fair! When you have to pass gas, I'd appreciate it if you'd go to the bathroom to do it! You claim you can't speak up because you don't have the strength. I always have to strain to hear you. But when you're on the phone with your buddies, I can hear you at the other end of the house!"

Among other things, Tina was still frustrated with Tom's drinking. But knowing it was a waste of her breath to say anything about it, she put this on her B list: "I'd like you to try to stop drinking. You're killing yourself. I'd like you to tell the other people to stop interfering! I'd like you to be better at figuring out when people are trying to take advantage of you."

"Don't use your whistle so much," Jean included. "You could pay attention to things around here that might need fixing. If I don't notice them, nothing happens. I can't notice everything and you just sit here all day—you *could* notice!"

Susan decided to include the following on her B list: "I think you could do more to keep yourself alive. I have several suggestions for you. It would be nice if you could keep yourself clean. If you don't take care of yourself, don't expect me to feel sorry for you."

Finally, Mary's frustration and anger resulted in her selecting this for B: "You really just dumped this on me. Now you expect me to figure everything out for you and to be happy while I'm doing it! It's not my job to be your entertainment committee just because you can't do as many things. Why don't you try to figure out something to do—and give me a break?!"

Category C: Things I Want to Say but Should Only Share with a Friend

These are some of the nastier things that, even though true, would be hurtful to our husband if we were to say them. We can give them voice, however, by saying them to a friend. This outlet is helpful, because it stops the energy of anger from getting stuck in us, where it can do harm. Some things are also quite embarrassing, even too embarrassing to say to our husbands. On top of that, we probably have some totally irrational complaints, because we are stressed, afraid, and exhausted. Sometimes even *we* know our complaints and statements are irrational, such as the times we declare, "I wish he would just get it over with and die!" Certainly these are hurtful things to say to our husbands, and yet they can slip out.

Speaking of Craig, Cathy declared these problems on her category C list: "He lives like a pig. He just has piles of papers and clothes all over the floor and half the bed. I couldn't sleep there if I wanted to! The bedroom smells so bad from his colostomy bag that I can't stand to be in there. He could spray, but he refuses to do it. It doesn't bother him! He thinks he's the only one that having no sex bothers. He doesn't care how it affects me at all. If he gets a leg cramp during the night, he turns on all the lights and doesn't care if it wakes me up—and I'm the one who has to get up the next morning and go to work! If I suggest anything to him, he gets mad and tells me to shut up."

Fran included these issues on her C list: "I wish he'd admit that he can't do things anymore. When he tries, he just makes a mess and makes more work for everyone. He isn't strong enough, and he doesn't think clearly enough, but he lets his ego get in the way, causing problems for everyone. He always says he's flushed the toilet completely, yet I come home and it's full, and it smells! I hate it when he lies about that. Then he avoids wearing his Depends and makes messes in the bed. Then he justifies it by saying, 'Since it's not a big mess, why should I wear the Depends!?' He complains that I don't want to have sex with him, but he wouldn't either if he had to look at what I do! Sometimes he has tubes hanging from ports in his chest that dangle in my face. Now how is that supposed to make me feel sexy!?"

Tina included concerns her husband wouldn't understand because of his mental state but that she needed to share with somebody she could trust: "It's just really sad. He can't clean himself anymore. He goes in and pretends to do it, but he comes out of the shower so fast, he couldn't have. Sometimes the women who help have tried to get involved with him and get money while I'm gone. I have to be very careful when I hire someone, because his judgment isn't very good anymore, and they can take advantage. He doesn't know how to protect himself from that."

Jean's category C list included these complaints: "I wish he could move his own wheelchair around. There are days when I am on the phone trying to take care of some business, and I have to feed him with his tummy tube with the other hand. I just can't do everything and still earn a living! Sometimes I am so tired, I am ready to die. My doctor said I *would* die if I didn't get more rest. I sometimes stop for a drink on the way home just to be able to face it again—and I made it a double! I want to take that whistle from him and stick it somewhere!"

Susan's C list included these responses: "I think it's really disgusting that he doesn't clean himself, even when he could. I could go and have an affair if he doesn't want to have sex with me, but I wouldn't do that. He's so damned dramatic about his health. He thinks nobody else has problems but him. Sometimes I just have to let him have it. I'm not sorry for what I've said but the way I've said it. I have no interest in ever doing this again. This is hard work!"

Mary shared these category C responses: "Mark has to get up and go to the bathroom time after time, all night long. It's such an annoyance, and it keeps me awake. I've got him wearing Depends, and that helps a little. And he always looks like such a slouch in his clothes. He doesn't care, but I hate to have people see him look like that. Why doesn't he care about his appearance? He's going to ruin our social life just at the time I think we need it the most."

Category D: Things I Really Need to Talk About, Know About, Have Resolved, or Make a Decision About

What's left now are the issues we are likely to discuss with our husbands. Here's what the six wives included in this category.

— Cathy —

1. I need to know what life insurance there is, what debts we have, and what money there will be for me to live on once you're gone.

2. I have no idea how my daughter and I will live once you're gone.

3. I need to have you treat me better.

4. I need to have you stop taking your anger out on me, particularly in public.

— Fran —

1. I can't deal with the sex issues anymore.

2. I am bothered that you still smoke, particularly in the bedroom.

3. I need to know if you want to be at home for your passing (if you have the choice).

4. I need you to come to where I am, if you expect me to hear you, and to stop calling me "Mumbles" just because you can't hear me.

5. I don't think it's fair that you expect me to miss my appointments just so I can go to yours.

— Tina —

1. I've already taken care of things, so there's nothing I need to know. And with his dementia, he's not going to be able to give me answers to things I would need to know. It's too late for that.

— Jean —

1. I need to know how to fix things, like the water heater. That's about the only kind of thing he can teach me now. Everything else has been talked over and figured out.

2. I need to have some time to myself, and I need to get more sleep.

— Susan —

1. I'd like you to clean up and come to the table to eat once a week.

2. I'd like you to make love to me.

3. I'd like you to share things with me. Tell me what you're thinking.

4. Because I'm being a wife, mom, secretary, and bookkeeper, it would be nice if I could bounce ideas off you.

5. You won't get clean for me, but you'll do it for other people. That hurts me.

6. Our house is too silent.

— Mary —

1. I really need to know more about our money situation. I want to have those talks with you, not with our lawyer.

2. I'd like to find a way for me to be here for you and yet still have some semblance of my normal life.

3. I don't like that you repeatedly ask what we are doing during each day and what time we are doing it.

4. I feel it's disrespectful of me when you don't shave or keep yourself neat like you used to.

Finalizing Our Discussion Topics

You may have noticed in looking over the lists that much of the angry tone left the six wives. Previously, their anger about other issues had stopped them from seeing things they might be able to change. Notice also that if we let too much time go by, as Tina did, we lose our chance to talk about, know about, have resolved, or make decisions about things that may be the most important to us.

Remember that you can have as many responses to each of the twenty-four prompts as you want. That means you may have many more items to put in the categories. I only included a representative sample for each wife, so your D list may end up a lot longer than these examples.

Because your category D may include many items, you need to decide which of them you want to discuss. You may start with easy topics and move to the more difficult. Or you may want to start with the biggest issue first. There's no right or wrong approach.

It is helpful to put numbers, in pencil, next to each item so you remember their priority to you. Or you can simply arrange them in order of importance, particularly if you're using strips of paper or a computer. This organization will help ensure that the things you really need to address don't get put off until it is too late. The topics of the six wives are listed in the orders they wanted to discuss them with their husbands. Of course, they could change those orders if they wished, and so can you. Flexibility is important.

The number of topics you end up discussing will depend on your husband's stamina, your stamina, and how well you are doing once the discussion starts. Because mutual respect, compassion, and kindness are the watchwords for these kinds of discussions, you may later shift some items on the D list to the C list, deciding instead to share those concerns with supportive and nonjudgmental friends. However, if you still feel you want to discuss those with your husband, it is your choice. This is your life, and you know what you need.

chapter 3

Communication Tools 101 (or Shall I Say, 9-1-1)

U SING SOME OF THESE TOOLS may seem unwieldy while you learn them, and you may not even like them at first. It is rather like learning to do a new gym exercise correctly—the movement may feel awkward and even uncomfortable at the beginning, but it quickly becomes the only way that feels right. Soon you'll wish you'd learned these tools years ago!

If you look at the twenty-four prompts, you'll notice that only two begin with the word "why," and none of the topics the women chose to discuss with their husbands began with "why." When we ask our husbands "why," usually it is a circular request for a change in behavior. If we say, "Why do you keep yelling at me?" we don't really want to know *why*. What we really want to express is, "Stop yelling at me!" If we say, "Why don't you pick up your clothes?" we really mean, "Pick up your clothes!" We need to say what we mean. When we do so, "why" will be out of the question, so to speak. It wastes everyone's time and energy.

Keep Your Viewpoint While Your Husband and Others Keep Theirs, Yet Still Get What You Want

Very often, people talk on and on and on about their points of view or their sides of an issue. Usually it is because they assume others don't understand them. Surely if people understood them, they'd be agreeing with them by now and changing their opinions or behaviors. The truth is, though, that other people may fully understand and yet still fully disagree with it. I am reminded of a very frustrating conversation I had with someone who kept harping on an issue. Finally, to get her to stop, I said, "I understand what you're saying—I just don't agree." With a look of surprise on her face, she said, "Oh!" and changed the subject.

We are never obligated to change our point of view to please someone else. It is perfectly fine if we hold a different viewpoint. And as much as we may not like it, when someone disagrees with us, that person has no obligation to change to our point of view either. Sometimes change takes place, but most times it doesn't. Nor is it necessary to make the other person *wrong* for us to be right. As one of my clients beautifully said many years ago, "Oh, I don't have to blow out somebody else's candle to keep mine lit!"

Here are some examples of how to handle the two sides of the dilemma—not having to change your viewpoint while not requiring another person to change theirs—and still getting what you want.

Assume your husband made the statement, "I hate peas" (or "I hate pink," "I hate tennis," "I hate chick flicks," "I hate putting down the toilet seat," or "I hate wearing a diaper"). After he says, "I hate peas," he tells you that peas have a bad texture, they roll around on the plate, they give him gas, they are too salty, he doesn't like the color, and on and on and on. He keeps explaining and repeating, hoping to change your mind so you won't like peas either or, at least, will stop serving the damned things.

It is really all right that he doesn't like what you want him to like. Ideally, though, he'll agree to what you wish. However, your goal is to create an Understanding so that your life will work, or work better than it has been working. So, you may say to your husband, "I get that you don't like peas—I just don't agree." An even simpler response could be, "Let's just agree to disagree about peas." Or, "I will eat peas, and you may eat something else." Or, "I'm cooking peas tonight; would you like me to cook something else for you?" Or, "I'm cooking peas tonight, and if you'd like something else, then you may cook that" (stated without attitude).

Change a Person's Behavior, Whether or Not They Change Their Opinion

Perhaps the issue is whether or not your husband needs to eat peas (like pink, play tennis, watch chick flicks, put down the toilet seat, or wear a diaper) for his health. You want to change his behavior, regardless of whether or not he changes his opinion. This is really an important concept, so I'll repeat it. **You want to change his behavior, regardless of whether or not he changes his opinion.** This probably should be your goal all the time. Do you really care whether he changes his opinion, as long as he changes his behavior? What if he still hates peas but agrees to eat them anyway?

To accomplish this goal, use what I call "I realize; however…" statements. You are not making your husband wrong to make yourself right. It isn't necessary. To start, always repeat the exact words he uses. This is not reflective listening; rather, this technique is designed to keep you out of the pitfalls that paraphrasing and interpreting create. Because he has said, "I hate peas," you say, "*I realize* you hate peas; *however*, they contain some nutrients that would be helpful for you." You may say, "*I realize* you hate peas; *however,* it's what the nutritionist said is good for you." Or, "*I realize* you hate peas; *however,* I love you, and I want to give you the healthiest food possible."

Depending on how important the issue is, you may continue in this manner until your husband agrees to eat peas. If no progress is made, ultimately you may have to agree to disagree. In this case, although you haven't won the issue as you would have wished, you've won several important things, including the following: You have dropped an area of responsibility; you get to stop wasting energy on the issue; you get to eliminate arguments and tension from your home, for both of you; and you can still like peas! You're making life work!

Changing Your Behavior
May Make It Unnecessary for Other People
to Change Theirs

Sometimes, it may result in *you* having to change *your* behavior, rather than your husband changing his. An example discussed in Chapter 6 involves a husband's decision to drive, even though he is impaired physically or mentally. He might say, "I'm perfectly capable of driving." His wife might respond, "I realize *you say* you're perfectly capable of driving; *however,* I'm concerned that you may hurt or kill yourself or other people." She then might say, "I realize *you say* you're perfectly capable of driving; *however,* I no longer feel safe in the car when you're driving, so I won't ride with you anymore." In this case, the solution is that she changed her behavior because she would no longer be a passenger in his car. She could have softened her declaration by saying to him, "You are perfectly welcome to ride with me."

A big part of being an effective communicator is being an active and careful listener. Often you aren't in the mood to do this, but it is worth making the effort. For instance, the wording on the driving issue is a bit tricky. It turns out you need to include "you say" in your response. I emphasized it each time I used it so you can look back to see how that works. You wouldn't want to accidentally say, "I realize you're perfectly capable of driving"!

Encouraging Your Husband to Say More

If you want to encourage your husband to say more about a topic, you can repeat back what he says. This reflective listening carries no interpretation. It reflects like a mirror, giving back exactly what it got. When he says, "I hate peas," and you'd like him to talk more about that, you may say, "You hate peas [pink, tennis, chick flicks, putting the toilet seat down, wearing a diaper]?" with a noncritical, somewhat-questioning tone. He could very well respond by saying, "Well, I don't really hate peas. I'm just tired of being told what I can and cannot do," allowing for further discussion. If you want him to pursue that path, you may continue with, "You're tired of being told what you can and cannot do?" to reflect back exactly what he said, using the very same words. Now he might say, "Yes, everyone always thinks they know what's best for me…" etc.

Don't overuse reflective listening, or he might come back with, "Why are you repeating everything I say?!" Most of these tools are good ways to get the ball rolling, but then we need to move to more natural conversation once the discussion has begun. Our communication tools should be effective, not annoying. Of course, if you run into a difficult spot, get out the basic tools again.

If you wish to share your feelings or thoughts, use "I" statements. Back to the peas for a moment: It is tempting to say, "You make me so angry when you don't eat your peas!" but it would be more effective to say, "I get [or, "I feel"] angry when you don't eat your peas." You might say, "I feel like a failure when I can't get you to eat peas." Or, "I think I'm not taking good care of you if you're not eating right." (Note that the last two statements reflect the most likely reasons behind our anger over issues like this.)

Although what our husbands do or don't do may be the catalyst for our feelings, the choice of emotional response comes from us. Before I created or used these tools, I fell into the same traps, although I'm still far from perfect! Long ago, I worked with a man who'd listen to me complain about something someone in our department had done, and I expected him to join me in my frustration. His response was, "Doesn't affect me!" That thoroughly annoyed me. But more than a decade later, I learned that he was right on target. Not only was it neither his nor my business in the first place, but I chose to let it affect me when I could have chosen not to, as he did.

Pitfalls to Avoid

We also need to avoid interpretive listening, because it can lead us on some bad tangents. Interpretive listening is a therapeutic tool, and we're not providing therapy. If your husband says, "I hate peas," do not interpret by saying what you think is behind that statement. An example is, "I know you feel like I'm trying to run your life and make all your decisions for you. But I think these things are good for you." He didn't say he felt that way, so don't put words in his mouth. He may just hate peas (or pink, tennis, chick flicks, putting down the toilet seat, or wearing a diaper)! Don't complicate things by reading more into them than is present on the surface.

With the driving scenario mentioned earlier, I could have responded, "I know giving up driving is a very painful step for you" or "I know it's very difficult to give up driving." Sometimes it seems like a good idea to acknowledge what might be in his mind, but therein lies the communication flaw: That would be attempting mind reading. He might respond, "Don't tell me what I'm thinking!" You might be wrong; for example, it might just be that he just finds it inconvenient to give up driving and isn't emotional about it at all. We wouldn't want someone guessing what's in our mind, so we shouldn't do it to others. A final communication tool to consider is language. Because we are the ones who desire the communication with our husbands, it is our responsibility to speak *their* language. To simplify, if you need to communicate with someone who only speaks Russian, you can only get your ideas across if you speak to that person in Russian. You need to figure out your husband's language. Start paying close attention to and making note of the words he uses. How would your husband respond to a good idea? Is he more likely to say, "It *sounds* like a good idea. I hear you on that one," "It *looks* like a good idea," "I *see* what you mean," "It *seems* like a good idea," or "It *feels* right to me." Or maybe he says, "I *think* it's a good idea."

Speaking His Language

It is helpful to speak to him using his language (see, hear, feel, think—even taste or smell, if he uses those modes) if you want to communicate effectively. You could say, "I have an idea and I'd like to *hear* what your reaction might be," "I'd like to *see* what your opinion is of this idea," "I'd like to find out if this *seems* or *feels* like a good idea to you," or, "What do you *think* about this?" Usually my husband, a retired attorney, used the "think" mode rather than see, feel, hear, or sense in any way. So I'd ask him what he *thought* about something. Often he'd respond, "I don't know." At that point, my reply was, "*I realize* you don't know; *however*, I'm only asking what you think." I stayed in his "think" mode, which resulted in an actual (eventual) answer.

Summary of Communication Tools

Although entire books have been written on communication, the basic tools I've presented should be sufficient to get you started. You'll want to review these again when you are facing social and family issues. Your communication tools will need to be really sharp to make life work in those areas. In summary:

✤ You don't have to make somebody wrong or change their opinion to get behavioral change.

✤ Ultimately, you may have to agree to disagree.

✤ To communicate effectively, be a careful listener.

✤ To encourage more conversation, repeat back what your husband says without interpretation.

✤ Use "I realize; however" statements, using the exact words your husband uses.

✤ If you wish to share your feelings or thoughts, use "I" statements.

✤ Speak in the same language mode as your husband.

chapter 4

Talk Your Way to Understandings

T HE END OF THIS CHAPTER presents sample Understandings for the six women. You'll see how simple they can be. Let's find out how to get from where you are now to that point. This is the heart of the process.

Knowing what you want to discuss before you set a date with your husband for the discussion is an important part of this process. Your husband may exhibit natural curiosity about what you have up your sleeve, and you'll be able to handle this better if you already know the direction you want to take. If you are vague because you haven't decided what to talk about, that response may set up unnecessary red flags for him and tension for you both. So if you're still not sure, work more on your lists. Once you've decided on your topics, it is time to set up your "date."

You should never suddenly spring the discussion on your husband if you want a good result. The first time you ask for a date, depending on your history with him, your husband might wonder what you're going to unload on him. He may be a bit defensive. If you think about it, you might be, too, if the situation were reversed. Never start with, "*We* need to talk." Besides being a huge red flag to most men, the statement reflects *your* need, not your husband's. Always use an "I" statement—"I need," "I want," "I'd like to," or "I wish."

Don't get pulled into having the discussion at the time you're asking for the date. This will be a big temptation, but having the discussion at this point likely will be less effective, because you won't have completed the final preparation. But before you try to make the date, it is helpful to review the "I realize; however..." statements and other communication tools.

Here are some examples of how it might go. Let's start with your fantasy response. In this one, you say, "Honey, I really need to talk to you about some important things." Then your husband says, "Oh, I'm so glad you asked. I've been waiting for the chance to share all this with you!" And then there's the real world!

It is best to start with a statement such as, "Honey, I need to talk about some things with you concerning your health and your care. I'd like you to help me pick a time that would work for both of us, a time when we won't have distractions or interruptions." At that point, your husband's response might be, "Well, what is it? Why can't we just talk about it right now?" You can say, "I realize you'd like to know what it is; however, I'm not quite ready to talk right now. I'd prefer it if we set a specific time. That way, you'll have time to think of things to discuss with me, if you want. Maybe this weekend we could take a boat ride, have a little picnic, and talk about these things."

Or, you might start with, "I'd like us to find a time when we can sit down and talk about some of my concerns and plans for the future. Would Thursday or Saturday be better?" Often, giving a forced choice works better than something open-ended, such as, "When can we sit down to talk?" Of course, a forced choice requires that you've already thought of a good time and setting: "I thought we could drive to the beach and talk there after the crowds leave. What do you think?" Your husband might say, "Well, what are you getting me into? I don't want to talk about those things." You could use an "I realize; however…" statement or just say, "If you don't want to talk, that's fine. I'd appreciate it if you'd let me share some thoughts and concerns with you anyway." You may only get this much agreement on such a proposal. Go with it! If you get an inroad, take it. Don't cut it off, looking for perfection!

You might say, "I realize you don't want to talk about those things; however, I need to share some things with you and get your input." Notice how this approach lets him know you value him and what he has to say. Or, "I realize you don't want to talk about those things; however, I'm really concerned and I need to brainstorm some ideas." Or, "I realize you don't want to talk about those things; however, I'd like you to be involved in the important decisions about your care. If we sit down and talk about them, I'll know your wishes, and then I won't potentially end up doing something you didn't want."

Notice in the "I realize; however…" statements that the husband's words are never changed, nor are they interpreted. Never say, "I understand this is difficult for you," because that can be an incorrect interpretation leading in a direction you don't want to go. He could respond, "Don't tell me it's difficult. I just don't want to be bothered!" Then you haven't accomplished anything.

Another possibility might be, "Dear, I'd like to take some time to go over a few questions I have about your health care. Could we set aside some time next week?" He might say, "I really don't want to do this. What do you want to talk about?" If you have really good communication with your husband and you have narrowed down your topic list, you might say, "I'm not ready to discuss specifics right now, but when we sit down, I'd like to talk with you about timing, location, and the way you'd like things handled." But you should be careful not to share specific topics at this point, because his response might be, "Well, what do you mean you want to talk about the timing?" Or he might say, "Well, just forget it. I won't talk about those things." When making a date, less is more. Rather than giving him hints, it might have been safer to say, "I realize you want to know what I want to talk about; however, I'm not completely sure yet."

What If He Refuses to Meet?

This situation is going to happen to some of us. How we handle it will determine whether we get past it to create the possibility for future discussions. Don't fall into the trap of saying, "You never want to talk about anything! What's the matter with you? If *you* don't care what happens to you, why should I? Don't you care about me? Well you can just go &^%$#@!$!" If you use these types of statements, you'll stop yourself in your tracks for this and future discussions.

If your husband refuses to sit down to discuss things with you, you can try a variety of responses. As mentioned above, you can say, "I realize you won't talk about those things; however, I'm really concerned and I need to brainstorm with you." Or the simple reflection (using his exact words) of what he says may get him to share more. "You won't talk about those things?" might get him to tell you why and actually prompt him to start talking.

Further, you could try one of these responses: "I realize you won't talk about those things; however, maybe I could talk, and you won't have to say a thing. What would make you willing to talk? What if you decided what we talk about? What if we only talk about one thing? Maybe we could do this with a third person—a therapist, your brother, our priest [or rabbi, or minister]? What might make it work for you?" Of course, don't present all these options at once. These are just examples of how to get things moving. Notice I've stayed away from the "feeling" words and the use of "why."

If the refusal continues, you might say, "Let me give you a few days to consider it, and I'll check back with you Thursday." Or instead of announcing a "deadline," you might just wait a few days for a time when he seems to be in a more agreeable mood.

If the refusal continues, you may have to say, "I realize you won't talk about those things; however, some decisions have to be made, and I'm afraid I'll have to make them without your input. Let me know if you change your mind so I can include you in the decisions." Or, on the other hand, you may have to say, "I realize you won't talk about those things, and I respect your choice. However, because I won't have the information I need to do "X," I won't be able to be involved with "X" any longer." Topic "X" could be funeral arrangements, visitors, or any circumstance about which he won't participate in a discussion.

What you will do, in as nice a way as possible, is remove yourself from areas where you don't have enough information to be involved. This may seem punitive; however, this is simply a logical consequence. Clearly, your husband is making a choice, and if it doesn't affect you directly, you can be glad to have one less thing on your plate. This is hard for many of us, and you'll understand why this is the case later in the chapter when I discuss enabling and codependency.

If it does directly affect you, there will be other actions you can take without conferring with your husband. These actions are discussed in later chapters as well. Most likely, many of the issues we are raising are things we've complained about to our husbands before, regularly and always ineffectively. We may find that when we back off, our husbands eventually want to talk about these things.

What If *I* Refuse to Meet?

Not all of us want to discuss things with our husbands. Some of our husbands may want to talk about issues related to their dying, and we may be resisting. You may be one of those wives in hopeful denial, and you're afraid to leave that safe place, even though your life really isn't working. If that is the case, at the very least you need to give yourself permission to listen to what your husband wants to say, assuming he is not abusive in the process. If your husband brings up a topic you don't wish to discuss, you could respond, "I realize you want to talk to me about your funeral plans; however, all I can do at this point is listen." If the issue is too emotionally charged, another option is to have him give that information to someone you trust and respect, and then have that person discuss it with you.

The Setting for Your Discussion

Whether your husband is ambulatory or bedridden, it is best to select a time and place that will support your conversation. The setting you choose will depend on your needs, your financial circumstances, your topic list, and your communication skills. If you're sharing how much you love each other and are talking about how your husband wishes to be remembered, perhaps getting away to a very pretty place may be a good idea. It is good to create as many beautiful memories as we can.

If he is in the hospital, make the room as pretty as possible, or arrange to use the solarium or the chapel. If you have really difficult issues, meeting in your own living room may work. This venue may provide more ways to end the discussion naturally, particularly if the conversation doesn't go well. Some people prefer to have tough discussions away from their homes in order to keep that space free of those memories. Some couples go to the beach or the park. I suggest avoiding activities such as taking a walk together. While walking, you aren't likely to look at each other and can too easily be distracted by other things. But if that works for you, do it. Some couples face each other and hold hands the entire time they have discussions. Others find it works well to have one spouse resting his or her head in the other's lap so the connection is close. If your husband is bedridden, you could lie next to him. You know your situation, so think about it carefully ahead of time and select what might work for you. Be flexible and creative.

Try to select a time when both you and he will have the necessary energy, and you won't have the distraction of a treatment or medication schedule. Do something to make the area nice for both of you. Add some fresh flowers or some pleasant background music to soften the atmosphere. Eliminate harsh lighting.

You may find that once you start this conversation, you'll naturally be drawn to a certain place for the next one. Once a location is established, a psychological "imprint" for communicating is created for that place. That imprint will make it easier each time. My husband and I had an imprint for our conversations on our porch in the evening before dinner. Conversations never seemed to work as well elsewhere. Conversely, we need to avoid a negative imprint. If it doesn't work in one place the first time, try a different area for your next discussion. Learn what works and what doesn't, and make changes accordingly.

Preparing for the Discussion

By this point, you've created your list of questions, learned some good communication tools, set a date, and determined the setting for your discussion. Now, if you wish, it is time to practice the discussion. You may want to write out your phrases and statements to practice formulating them. You may want to practice out loud while you are alone, except, perhaps, while driving. It might help to practice with a friend so you get used to hearing yourself say these things out loud. Susan suggested practicing with a friend who knows your husband. That way you can receive feedback as to what your husband might really say to you. You may wish to role-play until you feel comfortable. The more difficult it is for you to discuss things with your husband, the more you may need to practice. I'm not suggesting you memorize what you'll say. And if you think you'll do better without practice, that's fine too. You know yourself better than anyone, so do it the way you need. Remember, we're not after perfection. And even if you do it all perfectly, it still may not create the exact result you want. That's okay too, because you'll have other options.

Before you begin your discussion, you need to complete one more step: You need to take some time for yourself. Look at your topic list and briefly run the discussion through your mind. Then put away your lists and notes. You may get them out again to have as a reference later. Next, rather than bracing yourself for the discussion, spend some time getting yourself quieted and centered. You may wish to pray for help and guidance, meditate, or just sit quietly. You may also wish to take a walk or a nice soothing bath or shower. Do whatever is necessary to get into a calm, peaceful, and centered state. Avoid caffeine, sugar, and cigarettes, which tend to make people hyper. Perhaps some soothing tea or some water with lemon would help. I strongly recommend avoiding alcohol or drugs, as they cloud our thinking, exaggerate our emotions, and keep us out of the logical side of our brain. Although you are bringing up emotional issues in an emotional discussion, you need logic to work through to Understandings. Remember to breathe. You may even want to put a piece of paper on the table where you're meeting that says, "Breathe."

One of the gifts of the slow dying process is the time to have these discussions. However, this is potentially the last serious conversation we'll ever have with our husbands. This may be our last opportunity to raise certain issues. And, more importantly, these may be the words we have to live with as the last ones we utter to them. Remember mutual respect, compassion, and kindness for both people. To that end, I offer a quote from an Indian saint, Shirdi Sai Baba:

🦋 *Before you speak,*
ask yourself,
is it kind,
is it necessary,
is it true,
does it improve on the silence?

The Discussion

Once we are with our husbands, the topic and our communication history will tend to dictate how we start. You may wish to start with a prayer or moment of silence, if that fits. It can be helpful to start with some cherishing act, such as sitting and holding each other or holding hands. For some, simply sitting down and starting with the topics will be best.

You may wish to start by agreeing to some general guidelines, such as stopping at one hour to take a break; if a topic is too difficult, passing on it for a later time; treating each other with respect, compassion, and kindness; stopping all discussion after two hours, unless you both agree to continue; and whatever else you feel is necessary for your meeting. To easily create an Understanding at the end, one or both of you might want to take notes. For some topics, note taking will be helpful, yet it is totally inappropriate for others. Have tissues and drinking water nearby so you don't have to get up.

Because you've done all your preparation by this point, stepping into the discussion should come much more easily. Nobody is going to be blindsided, and you're both in agreement that some issues will be discussed or at least raised. Rather than getting hung up on a topic your husband won't discuss, move on to others. Discuss the things you can, and save the others for another time, unless you sense you don't have more time. Remember, you will have ways to handle topics he won't discuss. For instance, many of the women I've interviewed found the most common refusal came regarding discussing finances. Whether it is a power or an emotional issue for the man, it is a critically important one for the wife who will become a widow. You'll still need to do something about it. This is discussed in more detail in Chapter 6.

You have other options if he isn't willing to meet face-to-face. One is to write notes or e-mails. You can write notes to your husband and he to you, if he is willing. Even if you are able to discuss almost anything, notes or e-mails to each other still may be helpful. Perhaps you'd be comfortable tape recording some things for your spouse to listen to, and then he for you. Although these aren't the ideal discussion methods, if you still follow the guidelines and principles I offer, they are much better than no communication. Find a way to make it happen. Otherwise, your old behaviors are going to give you your old outcomes.

Closing the Discussion and Creating Understandings

When either you've reached your time limit or have gotten too tired to continue, take some time to compliment your husband for participating in the discussion, particularly if it was difficult for him. Thank him for doing this with you. Yes, I know you think it was his job to do it, and you think, "Who's going to compliment *me* for all my hard work?" You may congratulate yourself, silently, later. However, the nice comments from you will encourage him to participate in future discussions.

The Understandings we create are devices to make life easier—to make life work. Many men relate more to "things" than to emotions, so concrete outcomes may be appealing to some husbands. Review what you and your husband believe came out of the discussion. You may review things verbally, but I think it is better to do so in writing. Include a list of what you agreed upon, the items about which you disagreed, and a tentative appointment or date to meet again. You may include reminders that one person is going to find out about topic "X," while the other is going to check into topic "Y." Although this method may seem silly to you, or way too formal and businesslike, it is well worth your time.

The Understandings can be set for any time frame you feel is appropriate. Some may be for a year, some six months, and some a month or less. They depend on your husband's health and the specific issues included. You will find that, over time, your Understandings may need to be adjusted. Some items will be removed as no longer relevant, while new ones are put in place. If your husband's dying process speeds up or slows down, the Understandings may need to be adjusted accordingly. Be flexible.

Although you don't have to put your Understandings in writing, if you decide to, each person should review them. Putting them in writing and reviewing them allows misinterpretations to be recognized immediately. You may have thought you both agreed to one thing, but your husband was agreeing to something else. This is not meant to be a legal document nor a legal commitment in any way, nor is it to be thrown in someone's face with the verbal attachment, "YOU PROMISED!" Rather, it is a framework from which you can make life work. Again, remember that the main purpose of all this is to get your issues and concerns on the table in order to find resolutions—even if the results are to agree to disagree. This can ease your frustration and remove tension from your home.

Other reasons for creating written Understandings exist. If you have them in writing, you don't have to reinvent the wheel. For instance, if you've determined that you'll only have visitors on certain days and at certain hours, and somebody wants to come over, you can refer back to the Understanding to see what was agreed upon. You'll be able to say to a potential visitor that you and your husband agreed that he would only receive visitors between 10:00 AM and noon and that visits would be limited to a half hour.

My husband and I had been forming his funeral arrangements for eight years. We were in total agreement, but circumstances changed over the years. Each time we reviewed, we'd just go back to the previous written Understanding to see what we had already decided. Of course we could, and did, make changes, but we didn't have to start from scratch. I often found when writing the Understandings that we had failed to address some detail and needed to add it to our next discussion. For me, one of the most valuable reasons to have written Understandings was that I didn't have to clutter my mind trying to remember the things we had decided. That made my life work a lot better.

On issues where we simply needed to create Understandings about details, my husband and I often did it by e-mail. Yes, we e-mailed from one room to another within our home. It was an interesting form of intimacy. Because we had been doing this for so many years, we could remove the formality of setting time frames and making the next date. But we still put our Understandings in writing and reviewed them for mutual agreement.

As you go through your questions, and as you speak with your husband, you'll be surprised to find that some things are between you and yourself, not between you and your husband. For instance, you may have thought he was expecting something of you that he wasn't. You may have thought he expected you to eat every meal with him, but he was fine if that didn't happen. Or you may have felt he was holding you back from something you wanted, but that wasn't the case at all—you were holding yourself back. If that's the situation, it is a great idea to create Understandings with yourself as the six wives did.

Sample Understandings

Because discussions may flow in unexpected directions, we need to be flexible in crafting our Understandings. Below are examples that respond not only to each wife's topics but also to the directions the discussions took.

— Cathy —

Cathy's D list showed that her main concerns focused on finances for the future and the way Craig mistreated her. Cathy was not able to get Craig to agree to tell her about the finances and where money might be located. Their Understanding reflected that and how it would be handled: "Craig doesn't feel he should tell me about our financial situation. We used to fight about this all the time, and he is not changing his mind, even with our nice discussion. We agree to disagree on that, and I will not bring it up again. This does not need to be reviewed." Not bringing it up again was a huge change for Cathy.

Although you'll say that Craig "won" here, Cathy won too. She was able to stop some of her screaming. She never liked screaming, but she didn't know what else to do when Craig wouldn't give her the information. The Understanding dropped her stress level, and she stopped wasting her energy on something that wasn't going to change. It made life more pleasant and work better for both of them. To better understand how and why Cathy won something, imagine that your home contains a very large bell. You think something specific will happen if you ring the bell. Every day you repeatedly ring the bell, making an awful racket that reverberates through your entire body and the entire house, but that's all that happens. You notice that although it accomplishes nothing, the continued ringing damages some of the household contents, yet you continue to ring the bell. One day, you reach the point where you understand that this bell ringing isn't working and you stop. Imagine the quiet in the house and the sense of calmness that replaces the bell ringing.

Because Cathy's first Understanding stopped the screaming in the house but did not help her understand the finances, the second Understanding was with herself. This was another huge step for Cathy, because she usually didn't take steps for herself: "Because Craig refuses to speak with me about money or let me see the checkbook or bank statements, I will go to the bank and check all our accounts and bank statements to see what's there. I will check with Social Security, the VA [U.S. Department of Veterans Affairs], and any other agencies to gather all the information I am entitled to. I will go to the Legal Aid Society and find out my rights regarding what we own. I will find out how I can get access to all our information. I will review with myself in a month to be sure I have started doing this." She built in the time frame because she was well aware of her tendency to procrastinate.

To eliminate some of the mistreatment, another Understanding with herself read, "Craig says he's not screaming at me. He thinks I haven't heard him when I don't respond right away, so he calls out to me again and again. I will do my best to try to answer him right away and let him know I've heard him, even if I can't take care of what he wants right then. I'll review in two weeks to decide whether or not this is working."

— Fran —

Fran had many items on her D list. Her most troublesome issue was sex. Frank always brought up ways for Fran to be more enticing, while Fran had difficulty being involved in sex at all. On her C list, she mentioned Frank's demanding sex while he had tubes hanging from his chest. Fran did not want to insult Frank, nor did she want to encourage more sex. They jointly created this Understanding: "Because sex is such a painful topic for both of us and has been beaten to death already, we agree to disagree about discussing it. We'll have the sex we'll have and no more than once a week. We'll place the topic on our 'Don't Go There' list. We won't discuss it again." Note that they created a "Don't Go There" list, which was a very creative way to take care of their situation. Because that list cut this topic off from any possibility of further discussion, unlike agreeing to disagree, I would not have advised it. But it worked for them.

The smoking issue resulted in two Understandings. The first read, "Frank still wants to smoke once in a while, and Fran disapproves. We won't battle over something that will not change. We agree to disagree and put it on the 'Don't Go There' list." The second Understanding regarding smoking illustrates an option for changing one person's behavior when the other person's can't be changed: "If Frank insists on smoking in the bedroom, Fran will say nothing but will take another room in the house as her bedroom. This will be reviewed in a month." Here Fran employed logical consequences.

Hearing was a big issue with Fran and Frank, as it was for my husband and me. When Frank spoke to Fran from another room, he complained when he couldn't hear her answer. The Understanding they agreed to said, "If Frank asks a question from another room and cannot hear Fran when she answers, Frank is to come to where she is so he can hear her. Fran will go to Frank when she has a question to ask him." The second hearing issue was Frank's tendency not to wear his hearing aids. The agreement between them said, "When Frank wants to speak to Fran and cannot hear her responses because he isn't wearing his hearing aids, she will wait until he puts them in to continue the conversation. She will not speak louder to accommodate him. However, if a hearing aid is broken, then Fran will speak loudly so Frank can hear. This will be reviewed in a month." Both of these involved logical consequences. Perhaps because Fran is a school teacher, some of these approaches came more naturally to her.

It had been a problem for Fran when Frank expected her to attend all his medical appointments, which required her to miss things she had scheduled for herself. For this issue, a very simple Understanding was agreed upon: "If Frank gives Fran enough notice of his medical appointments so she doesn't have to change her schedule or miss something she needs to do, then she will go with Frank."

Fran wasn't sure how Frank wanted to spend his final days. Following their discussion, they agreed to this Understanding: "Frank will be at home for the duration of his illness, if at all possible. We will ask hospice to come at the end. We will meet with Fran's three children and their families to ask them to provide help when they can. We will also ask them if they can provide financial assistance to hire nurses when needed. We will review in two months."

— Tina —

As we saw from Tina's D list, it was a bit too late for her to get answers to things because of Tom's dementia. However, he was lucid enough to know what he couldn't do regarding finances. The first Understanding reflected that: "Tom isn't able to handle our finances anymore and knows it. He agrees that it is all right for me to handle these things myself. We will arrange for all the necessary powers of attorney."

The next Understanding was between Tina and herself: "Because Tom isn't able to clean himself properly, and it's dangerous for me to try to help, we will hire someone to do this. Also, because I enjoy cooking for him, I will still do a lot of that."

Tom's drinking was one of Tina's big concerns. Their discussion yielded this Understanding: "Tom says he'll stop sneaking booze. He understands it makes him worse. We agree that Tina cannot control that. However, Tina will keep booze out of the house so there is no temptation. We can review in a month or at Tom's next routine physical."

Recognizing Tom's dementia, Tina had to make some Understandings with others that normally she would have made with him. Tina created some Understandings with Tom's friends, children, and household staff. These involved their not smuggling alcohol to Tom and what would happen if Tina found any of them taking advantage of him.

— Susan —

Susan was concerned with Sam's "Howard Hughes" appearance and the lack of romance in their life, so the first Understanding she created with Sam was: "One night a week, I will set a beautiful table in the dining room. I will cook a lovely dinner and then get dressed so I look very appealing. Sam will get cleaned up and dressed for dinner for that one night. If Sam is able to do this and just doesn't bother, I will say nothing to him about it. I will then dine alone or leave and go out to dinner with friends. We will meet about this again in a month to see how this works." This showed she recognized other options besides fighting if Sam wouldn't comply with the Understanding. This made their life work. She no longer sat on pins and needles wondering whether things would explode, once again, into a big fight, and Sam didn't have to endure the explosions.

The second Understanding addressed her concern about not sharing ideas with Sam anymore. This feedback was something she used to count on and enjoy. They agreed, "On a different night, one night a week, we will sit, have a glass of wine, and share what we did that day. Maybe we will read the same book and talk about that. We will also meet on this one in a month to see how it works."

Because Susan had a problem with absolutely unloading on Sam once she started, she created an Understanding with herself: "When I am angry with Sam, I will decide which category my comments should go in. If they are really nasty, I will share them with a friend instead of unloading on Sam. If I really need to tell Sam, I will make a date and prepare so I don't *lose it* when I speak to him. I will review with myself in a month."

— Jean —

One of Jean's concerns was not knowing how to do the fix-it things Joe usually did. They reached some agreements while he was alive, and she created some additional Understandings after the fact—things she wished she had done. "I need to know how to fix the water heater. Joe will let me wheel him to the water heater to show me how to fix it." She knew Joe would be cooperative, so she decided there was, "No review needed, except to think of other things Joe can teach me to do."

The second and third Understandings dealt with Jean's being absolutely overwhelmed with all her responsibilities. The following Understanding remedied this situation: "Joe agrees that Jean needs a break one night a week. He agrees to have a neighbor come in one evening a week to be with him while Jean goes to the jazz club." Further, it was understood that "Joe agrees that Jean needs one good night of sleep each week. A person will be hired to spend the entire night one night a week, and Jean may take a sleeping pill. We will review in one month."

— Mary —

Mary was concerned about finances. She didn't know what to do, because every time she asked Mark to talk about them, he told her to speak with his attorney. She felt like she'd be going behind his back and betraying him if she did that, and she really wanted Mark to go over these things with her. During their discussion, she learned that Mark actually had little knowledge of the finances, because he had always let his attorney handle those details. That's why he kept telling her to talk with the attorney. She and Mark came up with the following Understanding: "Mark will not discuss finances with Mary. Mary agrees to speak with the attorney, regardless of her feelings. Mark is willing to meet again on this issue after Mary meets with the attorney so they can discuss how it went. This will be evaluated after Mary meets with the attorney. The next consideration may be that Mark will go with Mary to the attorney and be a part of the meeting."

Mary didn't like Mark's repeatedly asking what they were doing each day and what time they were doing it. The Understanding that came from this discussion said, "Mary agrees to write the schedule for the day on a board where Mark can see it. If Mark forgets and asks anyway, Mary will nicely remind him of the board but will not supply the information."

Mary felt that Mark disrespected her when he didn't shave or keep himself neat like he used to. In their discussion, Mark said that wasn't his intent—he was sick and just didn't feel like doing it a lot of the time. He wished Mary wouldn't mention it in front of other people, because it was private and it embarrassed him. The Understanding that resulted read, "Mary agrees to keep her comments private but does not intend to stop mentioning it to Mark. We agree to disagree on this issue."

Finally, in the midst of Mark's illness, Mary still wanted to have a normal life. To her, that meant staying socially involved, because that was "who she is." She ended up creating an Understanding with herself to accomplish this goal: "When I receive an invitation to something I know Mark can't attend, I'll ask if he minds if I go. He has always told me to go, but I just haven't felt right doing it. I will make use of the great caregiver I have and leave, knowing Mark is in good hands. To make sure I still get invited to events, I will have several events at our home and at our club. Mark certainly can attend the ones at home and can spend a short time at the club. I don't have to give up my social life." Mary is a good example of the wife who had been holding herself back but who realized she could change.

Understandings over Time

Most likely you'll end up having a lot of discussions. The process will get easier over time if you use the tools and follow the steps.

It likely will work so well for you that you'll forget the tools are making it work, and you'll start to skip steps. Then you'll hit a snag, and you'll remember that you have a solution.

Try to follow the concepts closely, as they are proven and sound, and they *will* work for you. But personalize the tools to make them fit your needs. Notice that each couple had a slightly different style for their Understandings. Some were very short, and some medium in length. You may wish, or need, to make longer ones for various purposes, such as funeral arrangements, in which more detail is naturally involved. The Understandings are to serve you, so don't create burdensome ones. Be creative. Be flexible. Do what meets your needs. Remember the words of Sai Baba and practice mutual respect, compassion, and kindness—even if you don't want to. I know firsthand that you'll be glad you did.

chapter 5

Comprehending
Our Emotions —
Life in the Guilt Factory

Our emotional issues are part of what makes our lives not work during these years. The intimate relationship we have with our husbands and the relationships we have with all the other people in our lives affect the private one we have with ourselves. That private relationship is what goes on in our head when we talk to yourselves. Our inner dialogue. The hotbed of our emotional issues.

A lot of external input affects us. Sometimes a *lack* of external input also affects us. Along with a lot of good things in our internal dialogue are the awful thoughts and feelings we don't dare share with anybody. The ones we feel pretty guilty about having—our B- and C-list items. Because of this, I call our inner dialogue the "Guilt Factory." We spend a lot of time here.

For the most part, we don't want to feel the way we do or have the thoughts we have while our husbands are dying. We'd be embarrassed if anyone knew what we were feeling, thinking, or saying under our breath. In the Guilt Factory, we seem to have the least control, and yet we judge ourselves most harshly for what goes on here.

I can laugh at myself now for the things I used to mutter as I walked away from my husband after something frustrated me. They really weren't very nice, and, at the time, I thought I must be really awful to think them. But these thoughts and feelings are just there and need not generate guilt. Actually, having them in our *inner* dialogue is part of what helps us survive, because they allow us to let off small bursts of steam and keep us from screaming them out loud or acting on them.

Sometimes we feel guilty that we're so sad or cry too much. We feel lonely, anxious, and depressed, and that doesn't seem right. After all, we aren't the ones who are dying, so we certainly shouldn't feel sorry for ourselves. We are irritable and find it takes extra effort not to snap at people when they don't say or do the right thing. Then we feel like we're being awful, because people are just trying to help in the best ways they know. We have a strong tendency to invalidate our own feelings or, at the least, minimize them.

At other times, something happens that really makes us happy, but it doesn't seem right to feel this good while our husbands are dying. More guilt. Of course, we'll have times when we wish this were all over and our husbands were dead so we can have a break or move on. *Enormous* guilt. As Susan said, "Just how long *is* terminal?" Sometimes we wish *we* were dead. Thinking and feeling these last two probably cause the worst and most shame-filled guilt of all.

Know that there is nothing wrong with these thoughts or feelings. They just are. That doesn't mean, however, that we shouldn't do something about them. You'll learn many ways in later chapters.

As you look at the fine dividing lines below, such as those between caring and anger or annoyance and sympathy, you'll naturally start assigning value judgments to one side or the other of the line. For instance, you'll think that caring or sympathy are okay, but that it is not okay to feel anger or annoyance. Not so. As I say throughout this book, emotions are neither good nor bad—they just are. There is no good or bad on either side of those lines. Any "goodness" or "badness" that exists comes with what that emotion produces.

We may feel so much sympathy for someone that we do everything to take care of that person, stop taking care of ourselves, and become ill. We may feel so much sympathy for our husbands that we do everything for them, causing them to become weaker physically and to suffer diminished self-esteem. We render our husbands "inVALid" as we make them more and more into "INvalids."

The word "INvalid" refers to a person who is too sick to take care of themselves. But if we use the pronunciation "inVALid," the word means not valid, null, void, or worthless. Many, many wives make their husbands "inVALids" on a regular and ongoing basis. The result is that sympathy, an emotion we consider "good," actually can have a "bad" outcome.

On the other hand, we may feel so much anger or annoyance at picking up after our husbands that we stop doing it. Consequently, they end up being more self-sufficient and feel better about themselves. So what we would consider a "bad" emotion ends up with a "good" result. As you explore these emotional issues, place no value judgment on them. You feel what you feel.

Let's look at what creates the strongest and least comfortable emotions on a day-to-day basis.

The Big C

Do you have a "Big C" on your chest? No, the Big C doesn't stand for cheerleader, caregiver, or cancer, although what the Big C represents has the effect of a cancer in its ability to weaken and destroy. The Big C stands for codependence and codependent behavior. The term earned its popularity in relation to alcoholism, but it can be applied to any behavior.

Once we are past the initial anger about our husbands' diagnosis, codependence is the single biggest cause of our deepest discomfort. It is the cause of our irritability, our anger, our excess work, our stress, our critical and guilt-ridden feelings toward ourselves, our fights (or verbal shutdowns) with our husbands over what they should and shouldn't do, our fights (or verbal shutdowns) with relatives over our husbands' care, the sense that we must do what others expect of us, and much more. It is very toxic. Yet, our biggest battle tends to center on not wanting to give up being codependent. We want to stay codependent because it feels right to us. It is a strongly engrained habit that has been encouraged and rewarded since we were children.

As you read the next paragraphs, you'll probably become annoyed as I question many behaviors of which you've been proud. Once you get past the annoyance, you'll begin to see that changing those behaviors will be the single biggest help to you emotionally, mentally, physically, and spiritually when it comes to making your life work.

Codependence is a term that is freely used but highly misunderstood and usually poorly defined. It doesn't mean that we and our husbands, in this case, are dependent on each other. Codependency, which is also called "caretaking" or "enabling," means doing for someone what that person should be doing for themself, which allows (enables) the person to continue weak or inappropriate behavior. We enable our husbands, and that hinders their improvement. It makes them "inVALid" *and* "INvalids."

Some women, consciously or subconsciously, enable in order to make sure their husbands remain dependent on them. The weaker the husband, the more he needs his wife. This dependence ensures her importance, gives her power, gives her job security, and shows the world how wonderful she is…the great, long-suffering martyr.

Codependency has many other aspects. We *know* how people should be, and we try to get them to be that way. It really doesn't matter who they are or whether we even know them. We genuinely think it is our responsibility to be in charge of how they act and what they do. We live in a "Burger King World": We want it our way, and we work very hard to make this happen. At the very least, it is our job to point out flaws and suggest remedies to others, just in case they might have missed something. After all, isn't it the right thing to protect everyone from making mistakes or getting hurt in some way?

And we are supposed to please people. When we're not running other people's lives, we are the ultimate people pleasers. We do what others want us to do rather than what we want to do, and everybody thinks we're just great. Their positive responses to us let us know that this "people-pleasing" behavior is good stuff! So, even though we don't want to do something the way our mothers-in-law suggest, we do it their way. They think we're wonderful. Of course, there's another side to this where our mothers-in-law neither notice nor care and give us no pats on the back. We run some pretty interesting internal dialogues when that happens! Either way, we silently steam, because we hate doing it their way and long to do it our way or not at all. Certainly we can't confront them, because that behavior is not nice and they might think *we* are not nice. We believe either silence or confrontation are the only options, because we haven't yet learned the communication tools in this book, so we suffer in silence in the Guilt Factory.

We mind read. We try to do other people's thinking for them. We partly do this so they don't have to and partly because we know they won't think of or come up with the right information. We plan everything they are to do, what to eat, how to function, and the way they should do it. And, we certainly *know* what's in their minds at the moment. We know they must be leaving their socks on the floor to annoy us or refusing to eat the healthy food because they just are trying to make our lives harder. Because we're people pleasers, we'd never want to offend them by asking what they really think or why they really do something. We think asking a direct question is confrontation and not part of normal communication. Instead, until we learn the tools, we'd use words that sound like we are asking questions, but we really are telling our husbands to change their behavior. For instance, we'd say, "Did you really mean to leave your socks on the floor?" Basically, we're responsible for everything and everybody. Pretty daunting work—no wonder we're exhausted. And these people won't change their behavior—no wonder we're irritable and angry. They won't do it our way—no wonder they make us feel alone in our thinking or isolated in the world. And they make us feel so powerless—no wonder we feel depressed. As codependents, our job is always about others. Again, pretty toxic stuff. And our job isn't about us. What a relief that is, not having to deal with our own issues or to care for ourselves. Phew!

You may be familiar with the song "YMCA" by the Village People. This is the one for which people form the YMCA letters with their arms while dancing. I always smile when it comes time to sing the letter "C," as it makes me remember the many times in my psychotherapy practice when clients shared how they handled a situation or asked if it would be all right if they did or said something and I, in response, smiled and formed the Big C with my arms. We laughed together, and they quickly got the point that, once again, they were being codependent.

As Melody Beattie, author of marvelous books on codependency, such as *Codependent No More*, has said, she really wanted to entitle the book *Codependent Not as Much!* Not only is codependent no more (or not as much) a more comfortable place to be, it is healthier for everyone.

I've worked hard on my codependency issues over the years. One of the biggest challenges of my husband's long dying process was that I was constantly presented with extreme and severe tests of my progress. You'll read about some of these in Chapter 6. I had been a very good student regarding codependency and was rarely codependent at the time my husband and I met. But now it seemed I really *was* put "in charge" of somebody — the very role I had tried to avoid — and would have to use the very behaviors I had tried to eliminate. But by using the communication and Understandings tools, I realized I only *seemed* to be in charge of somebody and soon returned to being codependent "not as much."

You're protesting now, saying, "Yes, but my husband is dying. I have to do these things!" No, you don't. You just think you do. You'll learn why in the section "My Way/His Way," later in this chapter.

Think about this. What if your husband could do more things for himself, and you encouraged him to do them? What if you didn't have to talk him into doing things your way? What if you let it be all right for him to do things his way? What if you used your communication tools to agree to disagree with your mother-in-law (or any friends, neighbors, or relatives) and still got along comfortably? What if you used your communication tools to acknowledge and to value the way your children say you should take care of their father, yet you continued to do things the way he and you decided? What if you didn't have to monitor everybody else's life, inform them of things they needed to change, or tell them how to change them? What if you realized not only that is it not your job to please everybody but that it is impossible? What if it were all right not to be in charge of every-thing and everybody? What if it were all right not to be perfect?

Can you see how your workload could decrease, your anger and stress could subside, you'd have fewer arguments yet better communication, and you'd end up with more time for yourself? Can you imagine how nice it would be if your internal dialogue were, "Not my job!" and you knew it was true and acted accord-ingly? Can you see how your emotions would no longer feel as tossed about, eliminating that roller-coaster ride from hell? All that absolutely is possible by becoming codependent not as much!

That being said, we don't become less codependent over-night, and we need to learn how to survive in the Guilt Factory in the interim. Often, while going through our husbands' long dying process, we have two or more competing emotions that we swing between. Because these emotions are so opposite, just having them is a source of stress, and we may wonder whether we're "losing it." Why do we experience such emotional swings?

Emotional Fine-Line Issues

To better appreciate why we experience strong emotional swings, we need to examine what they are. Then feeling precariously perched on a tightrope between them will make more sense.

Caring and Anger

Let's look at the line between **caring** and **anger**. Remember that Cathy said, "When I'm not angry, I'd really like to tell him I al-ways think of him as the way he was before. I know his mind isn't the same. I know he's really not trying to be mean to me." Under-neath your extreme anger, there is most likely a genuine caring for your husband. That's not true for everyone, as many mar-riages are bad. But even the bad ones had some good times, and wives likely have some compassion for their husbands as friends or human beings, even if they don't like them as husbands. You may wonder how you can be so angry with somebody you love or care about. What's wrong with you? The answer is nothing.

Our anger wouldn't be as strong if we didn't care or hadn't cared so much. It is our strong emotional attachment that makes the reactions intensify and makes this harder for us. Although we may look at paid caregivers with gratitude, we may also feel anger and resentment that they do all the tasks we find difficult and even have smiles on their faces. But it is easier for them, as they don't have the same type of relationship to our husbands that we do.

Or maybe friends or relatives come to help, and they do it with such cheerfulness. Again, along with gratitude, we may feel a little anger and resentment as we see how nicely our husbands respond to them, rather than treating them like servants, as they may do with us. The caregivers make it look so easy, and we think that it wouldn't be so easy if they had to do it all the time, as we do. This thinking is quite accurate. It *is* easier for them, and this situation is not only because of our husbands' reactions or because the caregivers aren't helping all the time. More importantly, the caregivers don't have the same emotional investment or attachment as we do. No matter who they are, they are not the wife, and the husband's illness doesn't mean as much, or the same thing, to them. They don't have the same memories we do. Nobody has the type of, nor the depth of, caring we have for our husbands. And nobody's life is affected more than is ours by their illness. And because our husbands don't have the same history with a caregiver, they may likely treat that person differently — maybe worse, maybe better — because their emotional attachment to a caregiver is not the same as it is to us. That's why our anger is so extreme.

On one episode of *Everybody Loves Raymond*, a thirty-something Raymond realized he didn't fit in with the twenty-something crowd anymore. He started hanging out with his father and the old men at the lodge, where he felt more comfortable.

His wife, Deborah, complained, essentially saying, "I got ripped off. You went from being an immature teenager to an old man." Deborah's comment reflects the ripped-off emotions many wives experience with the dying/declines of their husbands. Most of us anticipated a long and wonderful life with our husbands. Now we see what our husbands can't do. We see what they won't do. Our lives have been put on hold, and we can't even imagine the future. The future doesn't seem to exist. Where once ideas and plans and mental pictures filled the space, it is now all blank. We would rather be doing so many things now, but we can't do them, because we're caregivers. We're angry that our husbands may have caused their own illness, either directly or indirectly, and they still won't do what they need to do to be better. We are angry about all those items we put on our lists And angry that we can't fix our husbands and make them well.

We haven't had good communication tools at our disposal, so we kept our mouths shut, thinking we were keeping the peace. But we don't feel peaceful. Some women respond by getting into big fights and screaming matches. Instead of using either of those options, you can get the anger out of your system, your body, and your mind. I devised a healthy way for my clients to release their anger, any time, any place called "The Boulder Activity."

The Boulder Activity: A Silent Imagery Activity
for Releasing Anger
Sit so that you are comfortable and undisturbed. Relax for a few moments, taking a few deep, comfortable breaths. Then, while in a relaxed state, pretend you're in a beautiful woodland setting. (*Notice that I'm saying "pretend"—I'm not saying you have to "see" these things.*) You're walking along by yourself, and it is a lovely day. In the woods, you find a large rock or boulder. The boulder represents something that angers, annoys, or frustrates you. It is never a person, because we don't want to send negative energy to anyone. It can, however, be what someone has said, what some-

one has done, an incident, an event, or a situation. It is never you, because we shouldn't send negative energy to ourselves, either. However, it can be things you have said or done, or not said or not done.

Lying next to the boulder is a sledge hammer. Pretend to pick it up. (*Note: You don't have to "see" this either. But, if you do "see" this in your mind's eye, it should be what you would see if you actually did it, such as your arms, hands, legs, or feet. If you see your back or sides, you're observing the activity rather than living it. Merely observing likely won't be as beneficial, but you may start that way if it feels safer for you. Later, you may progress to living it in your imagination.*) You're not going to try to break up the boulder or even break pieces off it, because you can't change what has happened. However, you can unstuff your emotions. Many families have three unspoken rules: Don't talk, don't trust, and don't feel. However, feelings are neither good nor bad—they just are. We can feel them fully and release them from our bodies.

The nice thing about being in these woods is that they are the complaint department of the world. You can say anything you want. No one will hear it. No one will be hurt by it, and no one will talk back. The boulder represents the person's behavior, so you are not hitting the person. However, what you say in the woods is what you would say if you could tell that person off. As you tell the person off, be specific—"I'm angry at you because you _____. I'm angry with you because you never _____. Why didn't you _____?" Be sure you actually identify and express the issues rather than just swear at the person or scream in the woods. If you don't bring up the issues, you won't move through your anger.

It is critically important to say the issues in your mind while you hit with the sledge hammer. Remember, you are not just "doing" anger or "being" angry. You are "processing" anger out of your body to get rid of it. Although we can't change a circumstance, we can change the remaining effects of it by removing the anger from our bodies. Saying the issues in our minds gets them untangled from our emotions. Mentally hitting with the sledge hammer gets the physical effects out of our bodies. You must do both.

Sometimes you'll shed tears as the anger is released. Keep doing the activity right through the tears. Continue the activity until it seems like your arms are so tired you can barely lift them. Then end with a nice deep sigh and move to your relaxing place in your imagination.

Use this activity any time you know you are angry or know you have some anger issue. You don't have to make yourself angry before starting the activity. If you have stuffed anger, it will come up on its own as you mechanically go through these steps.

Annoyance and Sympathy

We walk another fine line between **annoyance** and **sympathy**. Without exception, the wives I spoke with experienced times of extreme sympathy for their husbands' conditions, as well as extreme annoyance with certain aspects of the situations. This is to be expected. Mary used to look at Mark and see a man who dressed impeccably, but now she saw clothing that hung inappropriately. She was embarrassed and annoyed that he didn't care about his appearance any longer. At a lovely cocktail party they hosted, Mark fell while walking across the living room. Mary was annoyed that it upset the guests and made them think Mark might be drunk. At the same time, she felt guilty about those thoughts, because he had Parkinson's and had neither the energy to take the same care of himself nor the balance to walk easily, and he'd eventually get worse. For all of that, and more, she felt great sympathy for this wonderful man.

Because my husband frequently got stuck for blood tests or for dialysis, he always had little bandages on his body. Often I was annoyed, because I'd find his little bandages on the rug, a table, or the countertop. One day I opened a package of lettuce and a bandage was sticking to it! I thought he certainly could be more careful and pay attention to where these ended up. Yet I knew what each little bandage represented.

Also, his arthritis crippled him and made it hard for him to get up from a chair. I'd get annoyed that he took forever to get out of a chair, particularly because he refused to get an automated chair to help him up. Yet it was painful to watch him suffer. I could hear bone on bone as he managed to lift himself. I had extreme sympathy for what he was going through and for how hard he was trying to keep our life normal by not bringing special furniture into our home.

Tina was extremely annoyed at her husband for sneaking alcohol. Yet she saw how happy Tom was when his "accomplices" visited. So few things brought him happiness during his illness, and she was sorry for that and for having to be the bad guy.

Cathy was always annoyed at the smell in her husband's bedroom area from his ostomy equipment and his lack of care with it. Yet she felt sorry for him, because one of his cancer treatments had caused this problem, along with all his other medical concerns.

So, yes, we feel emotions on both sides of many issues. That's part of what's normal for us now. And that's also what will sap more of our energy and why we need to make a special effort to take care of ourselves.

If you're feeling a lot of annoyance, you need to try the Boulder Activity. If you deal with your feelings while they are still just annoyance, they may not escalate to anger. The activity isn't going to change the circumstance, but it will make you feel more comfortable. It is quite natural to feel annoyed, irritable, and anxious with what we're going through, but we can fix that.

Part of why we're annoyed is that we're too plugged into the situation. The emotional split between annoyance and sympathy should come with warning signs, as it is very likely to push us toward codependence. Codependency causes us to step in and connect to a situation when we really need to stand back and disconnect, letting someone be responsible for themselves or letting somebody else take care of something. Let's take a closer look at that.

Stepping In and Standing Back — Connecting and Disconnecting

At the beginning stages, for those of us in denial, this won't be a problem, because we will be standing back and will be disconnected. After all, there's nothing to be concerned about, right? But once out of denial, we may have a strong tendency to jump in with both feet and connect with everything about our husbands—what they do and who does what with and to them. After all, it is their lives at stake! I think this is a very healthy and natural beginning response. It may not be welcomed, but there's nothing wrong with having it.

Unfortunately, some of us will deal with this dying/decline process for years and years. This brings predictable and natural emotional changes over time. With the passage of time, we find that our stepping in and connecting behavior either works, doesn't work, or works in some instances but not in others. If it works, we'll likely continue. The down side is that this behavior may wear us out, but we'll be so locked into this pattern that we won't see it coming.

If it doesn't work, surprisingly, we'll likely try harder. As mentioned before, it is amazing how pointlessly people continue to repeat the same ineffective behavior, expecting that some day it will work. In these situations, we may try so hard that we either get too angry or too worn out. At that point, we may reach the stage where we stand back and disconnect, but for the wrong reasons.

If we're too angry and choose to stand back or disconnect, we're being passive aggressive. We're expressing our anger by not performing necessary actions. This can get ugly and dangerous to the point of being criminal. For instance, someone's husband doesn't eat what she gives him, so she stops giving him any food. (Assume, for this example, that certain foods make him nauseated and that he is not capable of preparing food for himself.) She steps back and disconnects with a "screw you" attitude. Allowing a person to lie in excrement when they have no way to move out of it or to clean themselves up is another sad example. These are just a couple of illustrations of the unfortunate abuse, likely criminal, that unhealthy emotional states cause people to inflict upon a dying population of loved ones.

If you're too worn out to prepare meals and step back and disconnect because of that, it is not passive aggressive, but it is still dangerous. So if you've stepped back or disconnected for any of these reasons, you need to take a very *immediate* and honest look at your behavior and seek help from outside resources, such as calling 2-1-1 or 9-1-1, if appropriate. You can use the tools in this book once the immediate emergency has been addressed.

In normal circumstances, however, these types of problems can be added to your lists for discussions and Understandings. It is possible to stand back, to disconnect, and to let your husband be responsible for himself in a very healthy way, as you'll see in the examples below.

Mary stepped in and connected in the earlier stages of Mark's illness, particularly regarding his attire. Along with questioning him in front of people as to why he wore a certain tie with a certain jacket (using the words of a question, but really commenting that he shouldn't be wearing what he wore), she tried to exercise a lot of control over him, usually by humiliation. She could have been codependent and insisted on dressing Mark so he would look good. She also could have prohibited him from leaving the house if he didn't look right, because she was the driver. Over time, she realized not only that her behavior didn't work but that it was very unkind. She let it go, realizing Mark's clothing choices weren't very important in the whole scheme of things. That decision was very difficult for her, but she let him be in charge of himself, which he always was anyway.

Tina could have allowed or encouraged people to visit Tom, because it made him happy, even though it would have meant more drinking. She could have enabled the alcoholism. It would have been the easier thing to do, and she would have looked like a great wife and good sport if she had.

I could have helped my husband out of his chair each time he wanted to get up, even though it would have injured my back. He was almost 6'3", and I am about 5'5". The codependent wife would feel sorry for him and do that. And he might have thought I was wonderful to help, even at the risk of physical harm to both of us. In these examples, it was appropriate for us wives to step back and disconnect in the ways we did.

There are other places where we make decisions about stepping in or standing back. Some have been mentioned in the previous chapters, but many more specific examples are explained in the next chapters.

Holding and Separation — Moving Closer and Backing Off

This is particularly tough emotional territory. When we learn of our husbands' impending deaths, part of us wants to hold onto them so strongly that they can't leave us, as if holding on emotionally will prevent their deaths. We want to spend all the time we can with them and do everything together, as if holding them physically will prevent their deaths. We want to soak up their essence so they can't leave. This is a natural reaction at the beginning.

Over the years of your husband's dying/decline, the strength of this emotion will vary. As I said in the Introduction, during our husbands' dying process, the day-to-day matters of our role in their care, our previous roles, our self-care, our continuing lives, household management, sleep, sex and intimacy, changes in and strains on our marriages, and current and future finances are all right in our face. Practical issues continue as the living part of life goes on. The result is that these more extreme swings tend to diminish. What you'll find is that you'll get lulled into the ordinariness of his dying. I know that may sound strange, but you get used to it. As that happens, this process of holding on and moving closer diminishes. Yet the behavior will return when he experiences any specific or sudden decline in his health. And it may become very strong again near the end. Like all emotions, this feeling isn't going to be static over time, so don't worry that something is wrong with you if you don't feel that intense desire all the time.

Another reaction, which you might find more difficult to handle, is a strong desire to separate and back off, even at the first news of his prognosis. This can be very disconcerting to your husband, your friends, and likely to yourself. Two things may be happening here. One is denial: If we pretend our husbands are well and don't treat them differently, then they're not really dying. More likely we have gone into an emotionally protective mode, whereby if we withdraw from them, we can't be hurt by their deaths. This reaction is not unusual in the common course of relationships.

This response has several drawbacks. Although it might work well for your husband if he needs to go inside himself and isolate to handle his prospects, it may not sit well if he needs a supportive, comforting wife. That is not a judgment, simply information. The larger problem when a wife separates and pulls back is that she is using actions rather than words to express her fear, which is passive-aggressive behavior. To separate emotionally, we have to come up with reasons, so we start to identify everything that's wrong with our husbands. We find reasons to be angry and pull back, because we just can't pull back for no reason, or so we think. We manufacture a mindset in which our husbands can't do anything right, even if that's not true. We get locked into that mindset and aren't even aware we're doing it. Imagine what it is like in a household where that behavior goes on for years. Most likely, the husband will react to this, and then the wife will react to his reaction, proving the wife was right about all the things she decided were wrong with him. The good news is that this cycle isn't necessary and can be turned around completely.

Without a way to turn it around, husbands and wives do a variety of separation dances. As the years go by, the reasons to back off and separate change. A woman may have been totally supportive of her husband for many years but become completely worn out and incapable of staying close and holding on anymore. It is no longer about being hurt, as she may be emotionally numb by this point anyway.

A wife can physically leave her husband and get a divorce. While my husband was getting a heart transplant, I met another heart recipient whose wife divorced him as soon as he got his new heart. He wouldn't have been able to receive the transplant if he weren't in a supportive relationship, so she stayed with him just long enough to make it possible.

A wife can separate physically by moving her husband into a nursing home. Or she can leave the marriage while her husband is living in the home with her, simply by withdrawing her emotions.

Again, I want to emphasize that it doesn't have to be this way. As I said earlier, although you cannot avoid the fact that your husband is going to die, rather than having an ugly experience resulting in irreparable damage and regret, you can create a far different outcome. The possibility is that you and your husband can make it through these challenges, including the death itself, emotionally whole and with compassion for yourself and for each other.

Wife and Husband — Parent and Child

Whether we want to be in or out, close or distant, connected or not, the marriage as we knew it has ended. One of the most painful changes for wives is moving from the role of wife to the role of parent. In *When Someone You Love Is Dying*,* Dr. Ruth Kopp says, "In many cases the actual date of death on the death certificate is weeks or even months after the death of the marriage." Although Kopp may be overly dramatic in calling it the *death* of the marriage, certainly how we "do" marriage changes. As Susan said, "This is what it's [marriage] about — when people stay, and they haul each other to the doctor when they'd rather just run away."

You'll need help with these changing roles, as they take an extreme toll on you over time. Chapters 6 and 8 teach you more about how to create the possibility of a positive outcome.

The Stress of *Living* Grief

People tend to recognize grief at the time someone dies. Prior to that time, even the widow herself may not recognize that she has been grieving for a long time. But grief has an impact all along in this process. The moment we learned that our husbands might die, the grief process began. Although some say that the stages of grief Elizabeth Kübler-Ross identified relate only to a person dying of cancer and not to a caregiver, looking at them still has merit. The stages are denial, anger, bargaining, depression, and acceptance. Grief encompasses many things, and the topics change over time. They may be about our husbands' impending deaths, their pain and suffering, our pain and suffering, the death of our marriages, the end of life as we knew it, or the end of dreams, among other things. What you'll find is that throughout your husband's long dying process, you'll move into

---

* Ruth Kopp, with Stephen Sorenson, *When Someone You Love Is Dying — A Handbook for Counselors and Those Who Care* (Grand Rapids, MI: Ministry Resources Library, 1947), 151.

and out of all these stages, likely repeating a few of them several times. At times things may seem to improve, popping you back into fanciful denial—until the process begins again.

Susan shared that crying is hard for her. She's the kind of woman who doesn't like to be too emotional or lose control. But when she looked at Sam shortly after his diagnosis, she wondered, "How could his body do this to him?" From that moment on, she began her days by going out on the porch and crying. She did that almost every day for six months straight. She allowed herself to get it out of her system until she became tired of crying. There was more crying when he finally passed, but she had allowed herself the major release early on. To me, it almost seems that people have a certain amount of tears, and the sooner they get them out, the better. Holding them in isn't going to help.

Sometimes Our Emotions Surprise Us

We don't always know grief is there. I discovered that when I was helping my husband cut off a bandage. His skin was very thin and tore easily. On more than one occasion, the dialysis nurses had torn off pieces an inch square. To prevent injury, I carefully lifted up the tape from his skin so I had a clear path and stuck my finger underneath so the point of the scissors had to hit my skin before his. I didn't realize some skin was still stuck to the tape, and I inflicted a small nick. My husband wasn't upset, and immediately it was fixed, but for the rest of that day I walked around the house sobbing. Not just crying, but *sobbing*—very hard. I tried to hide it from him, but when he saw me, he asked what was the matter, as this reaction was out of character for me. I said to him, "I'm supposed to be protecting you—not harming you," and I bawled and sobbed some more. He was shocked that I was so upset by an incident that hadn't caused any real damage and was of no consequence to him. For me, I know it was the underlying stress and grief erupting.

I'm So Tired of Being the "Man"!

I admit this sounds sexist or old-fashioned, but the man of the house typically handles certain things. Although I'm mechanically inclined and can do many of these things, I became sick and tired of having to be in charge of fixing and taking care of so many things. Even when we hired professionals, they still had to be supervised, and it still took my time. Each time workers came, they tried to teach me to take care of something myself, such as the lawn sprinklers, the pool cleaner, or something for a timer or motor. Each worker would cheerfully tell me it was easy and assure me I could do it. In response, I'd scream, "*I don't want to do it! I'm already up to here with extra things to take care of!!!!!!*" But that screaming only was in my head, and I nicely thanked each worker and told them I didn't want to be in charge of that task. Although one of these extra duties wasn't bad, suddenly I'd have ten of these new duties on top of my normally busy schedule, extra duties caring for my husband, extra time spent on medical appointments — all coupled with the stress of knowing he was dying. So sometimes when they'd suggest I do one of these new things, after the screaming in my head stopped, I'd just go into the house and cry. I knew it wasn't really about putting the pool sweeper together.

Emotions and Words

Not knowing when our husbands will pass keeps us walking an extremely stressful fine line. Of course, every wife lives with this circumstance, but having a husband dying for many years makes it worse. As I say in the Introduction, every day brings a new challenge and an often-unwelcome change to life. Life is an on-again, off-again affair that tosses us about in the process. Although the gift of time allows us to prepare and to say all the loving things we wish, it also provides many chances for severe stresses and problems to develop. This can result in debilitating us, the caregivers, providing many opportunities to say and do things we could regret.

The better our understanding of our emotions and what to do about them, the more likely our final words will not be ones we'll always regret. Now that you better understand your emotions, let's take a look at some of the things that toss them around.

My Way Versus His Way

By now, you're dealing with some pretty complex issues. Having an awareness of what's on each side of them will help you understand why you feel pulled and why the pulls are so strong. Knowing you have choices, what your choices are, and the actions you may take will allow you to keep your balance, particularly when the pulls are the hardest. That balance is necessary to stay healthy on all levels and in all areas of your life. The previous chapters taught you how to communicate and the process for moving through discussions to Understandings as one way to create and maintain the balance. They also discussed your emotions. The following chapters will give you deeper insight into some complex issues and teach you how to take care of yourself as you face them.

I have divided the concerns into two general areas: practical and social/familial. Underlying all of it, however, is the dilemma of "my way versus his way." The manner in which we handle this dichotomy sets the stage for the rest of what we will accomplish. "My way versus his way" consistently is at the heart of our biggest issues. Certainly, we have created "our way" of functioning in many, if not most, areas of our marriages. We know from experience how that makes life simpler. It may be as simple as you wash the dishes and he dries, or he loads the dishwasher and you empty it; or, as I've heard some jest, he makes the money and you spend it, or you cook and he eats. However, that shared "our way" was likely thrown out the window when you learned of your husband's terminal illness.

Perhaps as part of the shock of it all, our natural tendency is to fall into almost a primal protecting-mother mode. What automatically develops is a one-sided Understanding that goes something like this: "I know what you think, want, and need, and I will be in charge of those things. I know what's good and bad for you, so I will make those decisions for you. You don't have to do a thing. I will take care of everything." Or it may be this: "Because I went to your doctor's appointments, I know what is wrong with you and what to do about it. I'll do more research and get every piece of information available to make sure your doctor didn't miss something, and I'll find out about all the alternative treatments as well. I will make sure you follow all the directions, take the right medications, eat correctly, exercise properly, stay neat and clean, and take proper care of yourself so you will be cured and we can prove the doctors wrong." Certainly these one-sided Understandings are founded on the love we have for our husbands and our desire to give them the best care possible — and for them to live.

Or our one-sided Understanding may be this: "Well, you got yourself into this mess, and you are the one who will have to deal with it. I'm going on with my life as it was. You're on your own, buddy. This is your job. Count me out."

I place no value judgment on these one-sided Understandings, except to note that because they are one-sided, they aren't really Understandings and likely won't work. If they were not one-sided and both we and our husbands were in accord, they would be perfectly acceptable. In the end, what we and our husbands agree to is our personal business.

As extreme as these examples sound, if you examine your thoughts at this moment, probably yours are pretty close to one of them. This likely is true whether your husband was diagnosed recently or you have been dealing with this for years. And that's perfectly natural. Throughout my husband's entire dying process, the my-way-versus-his-way issue was glaringly present in my home. Right up to his passing, I still thought I knew what was best for him. The important difference is that I learned to notice those thoughts and keep them in check, so I didn't act on "knowing what's best" very often without noticing it. Then I quickly moved to a discussion and an Understanding. Quite simply, one-sided Understandings are, and will be, the cause of most of our problems. They are codependent behavior on our part. The Understandings that we create with our husbands represent a new, shared "our way," and that's why they'll work.

So whether you've just learned of your husband's terminal illness or have been dealing with it for years, it is time to have a discussion and create an Understanding regarding "my way versus his way." It is never too early to have that discussion. If some time has passed, you're already making errors and heating up the issues based on the one-sided Understanding(s) operating in your head. But it is also never too late to fix things and to start fresh.

Jane is an acquaintance of Susan. She shared that her husband was recently diagnosed with the same kind of terminal cancer as Susan's husband. Susan recognized that Jane had tumbled into the pitfall of "We're just going to pretend Harry has something minor and go on as we were. We're not going to make a big thing about it." She created a one-sided Understanding that "they" would pretend it was something minor, although that decision hadn't been discussed with Harry. Susan suggested that Jane have a discussion with her husband, as soon as possible, about what each one expected of the other. Jane was in hopeful denial at this point, so it was hard for her to take that step. She waited until it was obvious Harry's condition couldn't be treated as "something minor," and then the discussions began.

When you are ready to start communicating, follow the steps that the previous chapters outlined. Jane could have started the discussion with such questions as, "Harry, we've got a lot of things to face in the next few months. I need to know what you expect of me. Do you want me to go to all your doctor appointments and treatments with you? What do you want me to be in charge of? Do you want me to make sure you take the right medicines and eat the right foods, or do you want to be in charge of that? Do you want me to find more information and try to learn about other treatments for you? I don't want to assume I'm doing what you want. I want to help in any way I can, but I'm not sure what would be most helpful. I need you to let me know from time to time what that may be. If you don't know, can we try to figure out something now? What do you think?" Just a few of those questions would suffice, but this gives you several good examples.

Harry may have had a variety of responses, including the fact that, at this point, he didn't have a clue about anything she asked. If that were the case, an Understanding could have been made to meet again in a month or so to see how things were going. By that time, his desires and their mutual mistakes probably would be more apparent. Or he may not have wanted to talk about it at all. On the other hand, Harry may have been in a take-charge mode and started the discussion and the action himself.

Notice the type of questions Jane posed. Rather than putting herself in charge, she tried to find out what Harry wanted. Rather than just asking what he wanted, her questions presented possible alternatives from which Harry could choose. Also, if she had really wanted to do certain things herself, she could have said, "I'd like to be in charge of your medicines, your diet, and your exercise. Would you like that?"

Ultimately It Is His Disease

His way may involve excluding you from the dying/decline process as he goes through it privately. He may have you involved only in certain parts or have you totally immersed in all aspects of the process. And that's exactly why "my way versus his way" needs to be addressed as early as possible.

You may be really annoyed and totally disagree with me when I say that ultimately it is his disease. Furthermore, I feel he has the right to decide the course it and he will take. Fortunately, you get to decide which part of his way you'll agree to in your Understanding. If he tries to put all the responsibility in your lap and you don't want it, you don't have to take it. If you want the responsibility and he won't let you have it, then you can do other things. As you explore the issues that follow, you'll see examples of how this works.

Cathy was several years into her husband's dying process when she recognized the presence of a basic "my-way-versus-his-way" struggle—and she was losing it badly. Her sleep suffered. Her health suffered. Her voice suffered from the screaming fights. Her marriage suffered, as the arguing put a wedge between Craig and herself. No matter what she did, she couldn't bring him around to her way of thinking and doing. Although verbal abuse had been a significant part of their marriage for years, sometimes it escalated on both sides to throwing things at each other, followed by days of stony silence. Issues had advanced to an unfortunate extreme, with no resolution in sight.

You may not have gone that far astray but still experience far more conflict than you'd like. If that is the case, as Cathy discovered, it is time to regroup and go back to the my-way-versus-his-way issue. To do this, Cathy went through all the preparation steps. Then her discussion began, "I'm noticing things don't seem to be working well between us. You've got your way you want things done, and I've got mine. I think we've fought about it long enough. Let's see if we can fix it." At that point, she brought up specific examples, such as, "I'd like to keep bringing dinner to the bedroom for you. If what I'm bringing really isn't what you like, maybe you could give me some ideas of what would appeal to you. I really don't want to start yelling at you when you don't like what I bring."

As they discussed their issues, Cathy needed to find out what Craig's way really was. She didn't need to give up her idea of how Craig should eat, but she had to be ready to stop imposing her way if she wanted the marriage to work. All along, as many wives do at the beginning, she had been operating from a one-sided Understanding without ever knowing her husband's side of most issues. Because eating often becomes a hot issue when someone is dying, I'll discuss it more specifically later.

In the following chapters, you'll gain not only insight into what's behind specific issues but also possible resolutions and Understandings for them.

chapter 6

Practical Issues

N OW THAT YOU UNDERSTAND that the powerful and sometimes treacherous my-way-versus-his-way dilemma underlies all your issues, let's explore those issues, most of which involve
the practical and the social and familial areas. Practical fine-line
issues relate to the basic affairs of day-to-day living. Social and
familial issues are those involving all the other people in our
lives with whom we interact, including children, other relatives,
friends, neighbors, clergy, and professional helpers. Certainly
these areas overlap greatly, as they also have an impact on our entire emotional climate. Many practical issues involve emotions
and interactions with friends and family. Social and familial
topics become part of practical decisions, and these interactions
have a great bearing on, and can even threaten, marital intimacy
and our personal emotions.

Unfortunately many more fine-lines issues exist than I have
room to discuss in these pages, but I have included the most
common ones. As you explore this sampling, you'll gain a basic

understanding and framework to work with any issues you encounter.

Practical Fine-Line Issues

The first practical fine-line issues you may encounter deal with the divide between your husband's independence and his safety or his independence and your safety. Rosalyn Carter, in her excellent book for caregivers, *Helping Yourself Help Others*, states, "You can take away a person's self-worth or sense of importance of life if you do everything and take total control." She continues, "Allow your family member as much independence as possible. Let go a little bit, even if you think you can accomplish a task better, even if it is painful for you to watch the disabled one struggle to do things alone."* She, as most writers do, discusses a "family member" and overlooks the unique dynamics a wife faces dealing with her husband. So although I agree with her in general, the independence of which she speaks crashes into many other issues. It isn't merely a simple matter of just letting go.

Mobility

Many independence and safety issues center around mobility. One enormous issue this raises is driving. It was one of the hottest issues in my household. Obviously this subject can create powerful emotional and physical markers for any driver who is about to lose this privilege. For our husbands it may signal not only a loss of freedom but also a loss of manhood and their ultimate decline and demise. Yet the risks are great, because an impaired driver not only can injure or kill himself but do the same to his passengers, other motorists, or pedestrians. Beyond medical, emotional, and personality issues, moral and legal issues arise.

---

* Rosalynn Carter, with Susan K. Golant, *Helping Yourself Help Others—A Book for Caregivers* (New York: Three Rivers Press, 1994), 83.

My husband's neurologist told him that he shouldn't drive because of his slow reaction time and poor reflexes. At first he pretended he literally hadn't heard the doctor's instruction. Following his denial, I took a stand for *everyone's* safety over his independence and reminded him what the doctor said. This discussion resulted in another trip to the doctor, who confirmed the instructions. It was such a difficult issue for my husband that he was furious and accused the doctor and me of plotting against him. He felt he was a good and safe driver who posed no risk to himself or to others.

So he chose to do what he wanted. Although he used a cab to get to and from dialysis, he drove everywhere else he wanted to go. Driving became the topic of a formal discussion, in which I shared, "I realize you still want to drive; however, you certainly would feel terrible if you killed someone, leaving children without a parent, or killed some children, ruining some parent's life." He restated his decision to drive. The resulting Understanding was that he would decide when he was and wasn't capable of driving and that I would say no more about it. It was an Understanding based on an agreement to disagree. I no longer had to walk the fine line between his independence versus safety. The Understanding allowed me to get off that line and have one less concern on my plate. In addition, one of my fine-line issues—his wishes versus my needs—resulted in my removing myself from the job of dialysis chauffeur in order to have some semblance of a life for myself. Previously my husband thought it was more convenient for him if I drove than for him to wait for the taxi driver. I, on the other hand, like Fran, was missing my own medical appointments and interrupting my activities to drive him to his appointments.

Of course, if he drove and I was a passenger, then the issue involved his independence versus *our* safety. The second Understanding was that I would no longer ride in the car when he was driving. He declared his independence, and I protected my safety.

Cathy did not have this discussion with her husband, nor did she realize she had options. Instead, she rode with Craig, and when she told him she was frightened by his driving, he told her to stop criticizing his driving and to shut up. So the danger and the arguments continued.

Due to the potentially serious nature of this matter, I called our attorney to determine my liability were my husband to have an accident. I strongly suggest consulting experts when you are up against these tough questions. My attorney offered to speak with my husband about it if I didn't get anywhere.

Using an outside source such as this may be a powerful solution. It may, however, be embarrassing for our husbands. You'll have to walk the fine line as to whether or not it is worth that risk—his feelings versus your needs. For some issues it is, and for others it may not be. As I walked that line, I decided that my need was met in gathering the legal information, and I could still protect my husband's feelings by not having the lawyer speak directly with him. In regard to the driving, I made four choices to keep my balance, three of which removed me from the fine-line issues completely. One, I wouldn't waste my energy trying to talk him out of driving, as, obviously, that wasn't going to work. Two, I wouldn't ride with him. Three, because of liability issues, my car became off-limits to him. Four, I could get legal information I needed and still protect my husband's feelings (balanced on the line). And the best part is that the atmosphere in our home became much more comfortable without the stress, anger, and arguments over this issue.

This is a good example of getting through a challenge whole and with compassion for each other and for ourselves. But undoubtedly some of you are thinking, "No! He won!" and you probably don't like the idea that I stepped off those lines. You likely think I should have continued and made more of an issue out of this, because I was "right." That would have been an option if I had wished. Years ago, I would have agreed and relentlessly tried to push the actions into alignment with my opinions. But getting off the line with an Understanding is one of the ways I learned to take care of myself, as described more fully in Chapter 8.

If you also face the driving dilemma, you'll be glad to learn that programs are available to test driving competence. The National DriveABLE program evaluates medically at-risk drivers. Agencies like this can be a great resource to take you out of the middle (off the line) of the dispute. Be aware that the test results are reported to the motor vehicle department and to insurance companies. Knowing that, a person may opt out of the evaluation. My husband never would consent to the evaluation, but because of our Understanding, it was no longer an issue.

Another mobility issue can involve deciding whether or not a walker is needed. Mobility brings up the fine line between independence and dependence. Although this is more your husband's issue, you'll find probably find yourself involved in the decision-making process.

Some of my greatest awareness in this mobility area came from working with my cat, Snuggles. Snuggles has a neurological disorder that caused the gradual impairment of his hind legs. Snuggles, like most cats and probably most animals, seems to enjoy independence and is very adaptable to change. Each time his condition worsened, I created tools for him to function independently. Once he lost his ability to jump, I set out step stools for him to climb. Eventually those stools were too big, so I created ramps. Eventually the ramps were too steep, causing him to lose his balance and fall. Next, special steps were made based on the actual distance he could climb and the amount of space he needed to regain his balance. He quickly understood the purpose of each item and readily used it, allowing his independence to remain intact. Being a cat, he was not insulted, offended, or concerned with what others thought about his need for and use of these objects.

That mobility issue was far different for my husband. On one side of the issue was his desire to be independent and to move about with ease, but he viewed the use of a walker as becoming dependent rather than independent, even though he often needed people to help him. Understandably, unlike the cat, he didn't want to show the world he was weak or to look like an old man. He felt more independent without the walker, and he didn't want to have to deal with the cumbersome aspects of it. So even though standing and walking were difficult, and even though he sometimes fell, his resistance was strong, and he refused to use a walker until two days before he died.

Using a walker is definitely a topic for a discussion and an Understanding. As those discussions start, the fine line will quickly change to the issue of your husband's independence versus his safety. You know his view of independence, but on the safety side is the issue of what happens if he falls and injures himself. Help isn't always available, and he could suffer a serious head injury or broken bones.

Then there's the issue of his independence and your safety. What if he falls and takes you with him? If your husband is larger than you, he could injure you if he falls. In your discussion, you should express this fear: "I realize you don't want to use a walker; however, I'm concerned that if you fall, you'll hurt yourself and I won't be able to help you. How do you want to arrange for help if you fall?" You could also say, "Because you could hurt me if I try to break your fall, I won't be able to help. And you know I won't be able to pick you up either." Ideally, the outcome of the discussion will be that he chooses to use a walker. But in the real world, he may agree only to use a walker when at home or when nobody is around, or he may refuse to use one altogether. You have several options. One is agree to disagree and let nature take its course.

One of my husband's retorts was that he was dying anyway, so he couldn't understand why I was so concerned about his falling. "What's the worst that would happen?" he'd ask. I have to admit that was a valid argument, although that's much easier for me to acknowledge now. A response to this argument could be, "I realize you're dying anyway; however, I don't want to have to go through the horror of that kind of incident." Perhaps with that comment, the Understanding might move toward getting the walker—or it may not. Of course, the fine line may continue into the eventual issue of deciding whether a wheelchair is necessary, but the process of communicating about it remains the same.

Tina was very concerned about this issue because of the size difference between Tom and herself. Because Tom suffered from dementia, Tina simply made the decision for him, deciding she wouldn't risk her own delicate back to stop Tom from falling. She provided canes, a walker, and a wheelchair where necessary. In addition, she arranged for more home care to help with more risky activities, such as bathing.

If your Understanding is that your husband will not get the walker and you will not jeopardize your safety, one option is to rearrange your environment to make it safer. Obviously this may be necessary anyway, but it is more critical when your husband refuses to use balancing aids. The *American Medical Association Guide to Home Caregiving* suggests many ways in which this can be done. It is rather like childproofing the house by removing sharp corners or sharp objects on which someone could fall yet also providing ample devices to grab on to for stability while moving about the house.

My husband and I used to take a walk in our neighborhood each evening. Due to his Parkinson's, he'd trip into sudden, terrible, lurching falls. Fortunately, he would fall away from me. However, it always took two grown men to help him up, which involved flagging down neighbors as they drove by. His doctor recommended physical therapy so he'd be stronger and could lift his feet more easily. He declined. Because the walker I purchased while I was still in my cat-fixing mode had been returned, I suggested we take his male nurse or some other large, strong person along in the event of a fall. But he declined this idea as well. Discussions followed, with the resulting Understanding, unfortunate though it was, that our evening walks would be discontinued. He was not prohibited from taking a walk on his own, but he chose not to if I wasn't with him. I would only take the walk if we had help come along. Because he declined that help, no more walks occurred. On my side of the issue, I was not only protecting my physical safety but also saving myself from dealing with the shocking and frightening experience of repeatedly seeing him fall and become injured. Following the Understanding, the subject was never brought up again, and I no longer had to balance on the line.

Later, you may reach a point when a walker isn't enough or isn't appropriate. One woman shared how her husband, because of MS, could no longer control his walker. He tripped, and the walker flew across the room, injuring their dog. The topic of obtaining outside help was quickly placed on their table.

Even if your focus is on your husband rather than yourself, you can see that being injured would make taking care of him more complicated, if not impossible. You'd have to get some outside help. But the fine line between his independence and your safety pops up here again. Assuming your husband is mentally able to make decisions for himself, if he will not accept outside help and it is beyond your ability to handle him physically, then you must do whatever is necessary to protect yourself. You could easily hurt your back, break a bone, or receive any number of injuries that would temporarily or permanently disable you. If your husband is mentally competent and refuses outside help, he has determined that he doesn't need it. Maybe he is correct. If that is what he has determined, then it is not your job to give the help. There is no need to put yourself in danger. That doesn't mean you shouldn't call for someone to help pick him up when he falls or for an ambulance if he injures himself. In my case, when my husband had minor falls in the house, I'd bring a chair to him so he could lift himself. The number of sleepless nights caused by my aching back decreased significantly.

You can make the home environment safer, as mentioned above. Another option is to have a physical therapist come to teach your husband how to fall more safely and then how to use things in his environment to lift himself from the floor. That will help him keep the independence he clings to. Ideally, he is correct about not needing help. However, if he is incorrect and you stop jeopardizing your safety trying to help him, he will see more easily that he needs assistance. He'll never see the need if you continue to jump in. That jumping in is codependent behavior, and this is an excellent example of why it is so hard to walk fine lines.

Eating

Another hot independence issue is eating. The issues of what, when, and how much are the tough ones. Often (quite correctly), we judge a person's health by their weight and appetite. In addition, a wife's value is still often determined, in part, by her ability to cook. When we see our husbands have a decline in appetite, it sets off signals in our heads and hearts. One, of course, is that the illness is getting worse. Another is that we may not be doing our job right. Maybe people will think we're not treating our husband well when they see him so skinny. We must get him to eat. And being the good wife, we must have him eat the right things.

Cathy's husband, who was dying of cancer, also had severe diabetes. Never believing that her husband would die, she fed Craig many supplements and special diets, to which he agreed. However, Craig still found ways to get sweets and candy. This sneaking made Cathy extremely angry, leading to arguments about whether or not he was trying to kill himself. Sometimes Cathy, in attempts to have peace in the house, would give Craig sweets but then be angry with herself. Cathy wanted to be in charge of Craig's eating, and Craig wanted to be in charge of Craig's eating. A possible discussion for this issue could have started with, "Craig, I'm tired of having these fights about your eating sweets. I realize you like your sweets; however, I am concerned that you'll go into shock and die." Craig would likely then have responded with, "Well, I want my sweets. It's my business what I eat!" Cathy could then have said something like, "I realize you want your sweets. And I realize it's your business what you eat. However, I no longer will give you sweets. And I won't try to stop you from eating them anymore. If you do get them on your own, and go into shock, how do you want me to handle that? Perhaps it's time we have a Do Not Resuscitate Order here in the house." Craig may or may not have agreed to that. However, the Understanding that resulted was that Cathy would stay out of the sweet-eating issue and Craig would be responsible for himself. When and if he were to go into shock, the agreed-upon medical attention would be sought. It may seem as though they had made no progress, because she couldn't change his eating behavior. However, the progress came in that the big and frequent fights stopped, and the household became a much more pleasant place for everyone concerned. Cathy kept her integrity by not giving Craig sweets, Craig maintained his independence, and both people got along better. With less stress in the house, Craig even became less desirous of sweets.

Mark lost weight but was pleased with his size. Mary, even at restaurants in front of friends, kept insisting that he order more food and eat more. She would tell him to take just one more bite. Mark felt as though he were being treated like a baby. Mary explained that she just couldn't stand to see him decline like that when it wasn't necessary. Their discussion, in private, then began, "Mark, I realize you don't want to eat more; however, it frightens me when I see you lose so much weight." Mark responded, "You make me feel like a baby the way you're treating me. I didn't know it frightened you. But I really don't have much appetite." Mary then countered, "Well, if you don't have much appetite, would you be willing to see if you could take something to fix that? I've heard some medicines may help." Mark promised that he would ask the doctor, but he wanted the nagging to stop. An Understanding was then created with agreement on these items and a planned review a month after the doctor visit.

You may remember the "I hate peas" example from earlier in the book that was given to introduce a discussion format (see page 42). It certainly can be applied to specific foods or to eating in general. You may wish to review that section for ideas.

Fran thought Frank made terrible eating choices, and he was becoming quite thin. She shared, "He eats like a 'man,' with no thought involved. Why can't he take it seriously?" He'd make his own breakfast, lunch, and part of many dinners. She used to criticize what he ate, and he'd just shrug his shoulders in response without saying anything. However, once a formal discussion began, Fran was surprised by the outcome. "Frank," she began, "I'm really concerned that you're not eating foods to make you stronger. I know I pick on you all the time about it; however, I'm really worried." The response from Frank was, "Well, why don't you put out what you want me to eat, and I'll give it a go?" For this to work, Fran had to be willing to select the food and put it out for him, which she was. Although this plan seemed like an obvious solution, they were so used to their old behavior patterns and to not communicating that they never thought to change things. A simple discussion resolved everything. If you and your husband communicate, these simple resolutions can happen quite frequently.

Fran and Frank built a review date into their Understanding. At that point, Fran noted that Frank consistently left certain foods behind. The discussion then began, "Frank, I've noticed you aren't eating bananas. Here is a list of other foods high in potassium. Is there something here you'd prefer?" He made his choice, and the Understanding continued successfully.

Jean wasn't as successful with Joe. He was proud to declare himself a meat-and-potatoes kind of guy and would rarely eat anything green. Jean would beg, plead, reason, and criticize Joe, but it never worked. Jean began the discussion, "I realize you hate green foods; however, I am really concerned that you can't get better without them. Is there any way we can get past that?" Joe announced that she should know by now that he wasn't going to change and that she should give up trying. Jean responded, "I realize you want me to give up; however, I'm not ready to. I realize I can't make you like green things; however, I'm willing to do something for you if you eat them. Every day that you have green vegetables and salad with your dinner, I'll give you a foot massage before you go to bed." Yes, I know that some of you may be thinking this is bribery. But remember two things. One, bribery is for something illegal or immoral, and I don't believe eating greens falls into that category. Second, as I stated before, in the end, what you agree to is your personal business. If Joe and Jean agreed to this Understanding, great. If not, they could have discussed it further. To me, this outcome is a much better one than holding to your side, continuing to battle, and never accomplishing anything while your husband gets sicker.

My husband and I also had the problem that his appetite decreased rapidly as he became sicker. He hadn't noticed how much weight he was losing, but he did notice how loosely his clothing fit. Since the colon cancer, he was very conscious of eating a healthy diet; however, he just didn't have much appetite. I knew that once they are in hospice, patients are told they may eat whatever they want. But he wasn't quite ready for hospice. A discussion between us began, "I'm really concerned that you're not eating enough. You're just wasting away, and you have no strength." He responded, "I know, but I just don't feel like eating. Nothing seems to appeal to me." I said, "I notice the things you do eat tend to be soft things and cold things. It seems you like noodles and things like egg salad. What if I make more of those for you?" He replied, "Yes, I think that would be good." I mentioned, "And there's plenty of candy for you to eat, too. You can get lots of calories by eating that along with your supplement. Would you like me to put it out so you remember?" We created an Understanding that resulted in my providing what I could that was healthy, plus additional calories (whether healthy or not) I knew would be eaten, and his feeling better as he ate more. Although at an earlier time both of us might have been appalled by such a diet, the Understanding was that this was the most appropriate plan for this circumstance. Eventually when hospice became involved, diet became a nonissue, ice cream was added to the supplement, and any type of food that was appealing was provided.

Cleanliness, Neatness, and Dressing

This is another major issue for several reasons. As our husbands enter and progress through their dying/declines, certain behavioral changes occur. One side effect of many conditions, as well as knowing the condition is terminal, is depression. Susan found this was the case with Sam, who always had been extremely stylish and careful about his appearance. You can see her complaints in Chapter 4, "Talk Your Way to Understandings," along with the resolution to them. Shortly after being diagnosed, Sam didn't want to bother showering, shaving, or getting dressed. On the days he did dress, he didn't care what he put on, how it looked, or how it smelled. Often he'd just stay in his pajamas, even though he still was healthy enough to be up, dressed, and functioning pretty normally. Sometimes he would get dressed for company or to go out, but he never would bother for Susan. Over time, he dressed less and less well, even for others. Susan begged, fought, and tried everything to get him to get clean himself and to dress neatly. Of course, none of that worked. Over time, Susan backed off from this issue and let Sam be in charge of himself.

Other men, perhaps as another side of depression, become rebellious. They decide to stop dressing to please others and only take care of themselves as they wish. Some decide to let their hair grow, maybe into ponytails, or they grow beards as sort of a "f*** you" response to the world and their situation. Maybe they finally get those Harleys as well.

In the two situations above, the discussion would be, "Honey, I realize you're not getting cleaned up and dressed anymore; however, I'm really bothered by that. I feel like you don't care about me or us anymore." Notice that the wording does not start by assuming a reason he doesn't get clean or dressed. It doesn't say, "I know you are very depressed" or "I know you're really angry about being sick." It starts with the simple fact of what you observe: My husband isn't getting cleaned up or dressed. It is very important to start this way in order to keep the discussion from ending up on a different topic. But if you really want to discuss your husband's emotions, you could begin, "I notice you aren't getting cleaned up or dressed anymore. I'm concerned about how you're doing emotionally. I wouldn't be surprised if you've got some pretty strong feelings about the cancer. If you want to talk about it, I'd be glad to listen." He may not want to talk about it, but showing this understanding may be helpful. It may not change the cleanliness or dressing situation, but knowing that you understand or are trying to may give your husband a little peace. Remember, in our preparation for a discussion, it is important to know what we really want to discuss and what we hope to accomplish.

Mary always was concerned about Mark's appearance, even before he became ill. She usually bought his clothes for him, insisted on the proper tailoring, and selected which items would be worn together. Mark was quite used to this routine after their many years of marriage. Once his illness was progressing and he cared even less about how he dressed, a discussion between Mary and Mark went something like this: "Mark, I really think you haven't been dressing as well as you could. It's really important to me that you look your best even though you're sick. I'm going to check you more carefully before we go out. Will that bother you?" Mark replied, "Mary, if you didn't do that, you wouldn't be Mary. Just don't get angry if I ignore what you say." This created an interesting Understanding. It was almost an agreement to disagree, yet it allowed each person's behavior to continue as it had been. Understandings come in many forms.

At some point, most men in their dying/declines cease to be able to take care of themselves. This situation places an extra burden on their wives. It can be very difficult emotionally, as it is another marker that our husbands are closer to death. Although this is an expected phase in the dying/decline, it also creates a shift from the role of wife to that of caretaking mother. In *When Someone You Love Is Dying*, Dr. Ruth Kopp shares some sensitive observations about these changes. "The well partner 'mothers' the sick one—cooking for him, caring for him, dressing and undressing him," she states, "[and] sometimes bathing him—assuming the duties that a mother undertakes for a small child."* Even though this behavior is predictable, discussions are necessary to determine the expectations and desires of our husbands and ourselves so no one-sided Understandings develop. Just because we want to perform a certain task (clean him, dress him, feed him) doesn't mean our husbands wish that to be done at all or for us to be the one to do it. And even if your husband wishes you to perform these tasks, that doesn't mean you have to do them. If you do not wish to, then the discussion needs to include another way to accomplish those tasks.

* Ruth Kopp, with Stephen Sorenson, *When Someone You Love Is Dying—A Handbook for Counselors and Those Who Care* (Grand Rapids, MI: Ministry Resources Library, 1947), 151.

Frank wanted Fran to do it all. He thought it was just great that she would give him all that special care. He felt so nurtured by it. Fran, however, still worked, so she didn't have a lot of extra time or energy. She did want to do certain things for him, such as help clean him and arrange for the food under their new Understanding. But Frank began to demand more and more from her, so another discussion ensued: "Frank, I realize you'd like me to do everything; however, I just don't have the energy to do it all. I know you don't like having strangers in the house, so whom do you think we can ask to help?" Frank responded, "Well, you just don't care enough about me. I don't want anyone else but you doing these things for me. They are too private. I don't want other people to see me this way or to have to clean up my messes. I need you to do that so other people don't know." Fran continued, "I realize you need me to do these things so other people don't know. However, it's impossible for me to do it all. If I get sick and can't do anything, then what will you do?" Fran then offered other alternatives, and, if none were accepted, she would only do what she could. She didn't push beyond her limits just because he wanted her to do it all. When Frank saw that Fran followed through on what she said, he agreed to have additional helpers.

Toilet Issues

Unfortunately, leaving the toilet seat up or not flushing the toilet after use becomes the least of the problems in this arena, because the more troublesome issues of urinary and bowel incontinence are common outcomes of illness and medications. An important discussion, therefore, revolves around using adult protective underwear. It is an issue of protecting our husbands' clothing, the car seat, restaurant chairs, and our partners' egos in public. In bed, the better the protection they have, the cleaner and more comfortable they'll stay. With protective clothing, any mishap will be smaller, easier, and faster to clean up. However, I haven't yet heard of a husband volunteering to wear the protective briefs. Adult protection isn't as big an issue for women, as they are more accustomed to using sanitary protection. But therein lies part of the problem for men: At some level, they think of this as not only babylike but also feminine.

Cathy had to take a rather strong stand with Craig early on. She regularly slept in a recliner in the living room, not only because the bedroom usually smelled so terrible but also because Craig kept so many things piled on the bed that there wasn't room for her. He refused to wear special underwear, yet he had frequent mishaps in bed. He still was able to take care of himself, which was an important fact in this scenario. Cathy had the following discussion with him: "Craig, I realize you won't wear your pants to bed. However, after I wash these sheets from last night, I will only change your sheets once a week. So if you have an accident during the night, I will not clean it up." Craig's responded, "Well, we'll see about that!" as he knew Cathy often became angry and then gave in. Knowing Craig's usual stubbornness, she put extra protection on the mattress just in case. Craig didn't wear his protective pants and had an accident, and the mess stayed for two days. He wouldn't change his sheets. After two nights, Cathy couldn't stand it, so she cleaned it up and made her announcement again. After several tries, including leaving the sheets a mess for up to three days, Craig gave in and wore the protective garments. When he did, the evenings and mornings were better for both of them. Notice that in this circumstance, Craig still had the option to do what he wished. He could go without protective garments, and he could clean his own sheets. He wasn't being forced to wear the pants, nor was he being forced to lie in his excrement. Of course, if someone were unable to take care of themselves, the option Cathy chose would be out of the question. But in that case, the caretaker likely would be able to just put the garment on the sick person.

Other related issues involve medication, medical treatments, exercise, and outside help. The examples above provide a format for dealing with any and all of these issues.

Financial and Legal Matters

Another very practical consideration involves his feelings versus your financial and legal needs. Let me begin by emphasizing that I am not giving legal or financial advice. It is always best to check with your attorney or financial adviser, although that in itself is a difficult issue for many women, as you'll see. Here are some issues to consider:

- 🌿 Are possessions (house, car, boat, motorcycle, motor home) in both names or will you lose them when your husband dies?
- 🌿 Has a will been drawn up?
- 🌿 Are you a beneficiary in the will or does the money go to other people?
- 🌿 Where are the legal and financial documents located?
- 🌿 Has your husband promised things in your home to other people?
- 🌿 Do other people already own things in your home?
- 🌿 Are any items in your home financed?
- 🌿 Has your husband defaulted on payments since he's been sick?
- 🌿 Does he have life insurance?
- 🌿 Are you the beneficiary?
- 🌿 Do you have mortgage insurance to pay off your home when he dies?
- 🌿 Has a trust been established?
- 🌿 How will it affect you if it has?
- 🌿 Does he have a pension that will go to you?

- Are death benefits going to you?
- Will you have to assume debt that your husband accumulated in both names?
- Will you be held accountable for financial obligations or debts that your husband incurred?
- Do you have health insurance to cover you (and your children) when he dies?
- Are you eligible to continue your husband's health insurance for yourself once he dies?
- Do you have money to pay remaining medical bills when he dies?
- Is money set aside for or does an insurance policy cover funeral or burial expenses?
- Which payments will you have to take over (mortgage, car, gasoline, car repair, electricity, phone, insurance, maintenance, home repairs, service people, real estate tax, income tax, association fees, club dues, charitable donations, pet care)?
- Which insurance policies do you now have to take over the payments for (house, car, etc.)?

There are even more issues than I have raised about which you need to make yourself aware and informed. Without specific knowledge, you can be vulnerable on many levels.

Sometimes a husband is anxious to take care of these matters with his wife. That was the case with my husband. Because we had a history of frequent discussions, this topic was easy for us. Every aspect was presented in great detail to be sure I fully understood not only what documents, insurance, and monies existed and their locations but also what to do with all of it, including who was to receive what, when, and how. Because he had a controlling personality, he tried to make sure things would be done exactly the way he wanted. I heard and learned more than I cared to, but I took it all in just in case.

Some women do not want to hear anything about finances and legalities. Fran was such a person. She never wanted to learn about the family finances. Her skills were in teaching and in raising a family. Money was Frank's department. Although I think Fran was unwise to miss the opportunity, if Frank brought up the subject and she didn't want to discuss it, she could have said, "Frank, I realize you want to teach me all these financial things; however, I really don't want to learn about them. I want to think you'll keep living, and I just won't need to know." At this point, either Frank could have tried to convince her, or they could have come up with an option such as this: "Frank, I realize you want to teach me all these financial things; however, I really don't want to learn about it. If you think it's really that important, why don't you give all the information to _____ (our attorney/our accountant/your brother/my sister/etc.)? If I ever need to know about it, I will ask them." Frank may or may not agree to an Understanding of this nature, but it is a reasonable solution.

Some husbands are uncomfortable discussing these issues, because they don't want to think about their imminent death. Mark was such a husband, yet he had seen to it that everything was in order for his wife. Mary, however, was frustrated, because every time she asked about their finances, he'd say, "Just ask my attorney," and she felt guilty doing that. She felt like she was going behind his back. But Mary had some options, one of which was to create the Understanding described earlier. Another was to accept the fact that because Mark had said to ask the attorney, she had no reason to feel guilty. But if her real issue was that she wanted him to discuss it with her, she could have said, "Mark, I'm really glad you've taken care of things so well for me. I realize you want me to ask your attorney to explain things; however, I feel uncomfortable doing that. If you were to go with me and sit there while she explains, I think I'd feel better about it.

Would you please do that with me?" Mark might have responded that he'd be willing to do that, or he might have said, "No, Mary. That's what I have an attorney for. That's exactly the kind of thing I pay her to do!"

Another option for Mary would be to say: "Mark, I realize you want me to talk to your attorney about the finances; however, I don't really know what to ask when I see her. Perhaps you could give me some ideas of things to ask before I go." Or, "Mark, I realize you want me to talk to your attorney about finances; however, it feels so impersonal doing it that way. What if you explain things to me first? Then I can go to her if I still have questions."

Susan and Sam had some different financial issues. She was easily able to get the information she needed about future finances. In doing that, she also figured out that they would be better off financially if they were to move out of the house they owned. Because his illness came at a time before investments or pensions were built up to fall back on, money was tight. Whenever she would raise her concerns, he would either act indignant and insulted that she could question how he spent money "at a time like *this*," or he would simply refuse to discuss it. In that situation, Susan's approach could have been: "Sam, I realize you don't want me to bring up money at a time like *this*; however, I think if we sell the house now, we would have the money to provide better care for you. We could have more nurses and assistants to help with things—all the things that insurance won't pay for. I don't mind sacrificing and moving into something smaller. It's important to me that we provide good care for you without running out of money in the process." Sam may have then responded by saying, "I'm not moving. I'm the one here who's dying and I'm not going to start making changes now!" Susan then could have said, "I realize you're the one dying and I wish you weren't. However, I'm not dying, and living this way is hurting what's left of our marriage. We're both affected by these finances, and I think we can be much happier if we simplify our lives." Even though Sam may have disagreed, Susan could still have explored possibilities. Perhaps some residential option would have appealed to his taste. She could have shown him residential information along with actual dollar amounts that would be freed up by the move. On the other hand, their home was in Sam's name, so the ultimate authority for making a decision rested with him. To avoid continual conflict, their Understanding was to agree to disagree, leaving Susan sitting on an uncomfortable fine line. However, the beauty of this arrangement was that the arguments on this topic stopped, and the couple was able to have a more peaceful household. Susan had the option of trying again at a later time if she saw the money situation become more severe. At that point, she may or may not have been able to get a different response from Sam. Additionally, because sitting on that fine line was uncomfortable, Susan needed to do more self-care.

Tina had a long history of being involved with the family finances, so this was a nonissue in her household. Tom had his affairs well in order, and Tina knew exactly what needed to be done and how to do it.

Some husbands are extremely controlling and, for any number of reasons, don't want their wives to know anything. Maybe they have a lot of money they don't want their wives to know about, maybe they have been doing something less than desirable and losing money, or maybe they don't have any money and they are embarrassed. Cathy and Craig represent this controlling group well, and their situation is one that is all too common for far too many women. Essentially, Craig didn't want Cathy to have access to the finances, and she went along with that. On numerous occasions, she asked Craig what money they had. She knew at one point they had had a decent amount of money, but he had wasted it on unsuccessful ventures. Household finances were always a problem. Even though she was seventy, she still had to work to make ends meet. Their adult daughter lived with them and contributed to the finances, but it still wasn't enough. Cathy had no idea how much money they had, no idea if they had any insurance or savings, no idea where any legal papers might be kept, and no idea how she would live once Craig passed on.

She said, "I never really had any trouble talking to him or saying what I wanted to say, and I never held anything back. I was just frustrated, because I knew what I would be facing after he was gone. But it bothered me that it didn't seem to bother him, and he never brought anything up." Unfortunately, Cathy had been getting beaten down for so long that she didn't realize her communication method wasn't working. She would yell at Craig for what he hadn't done, but she never got any answers. After he died, she searched for things, finding little information, no money, and a lot of debt. Yet Cathy could have taken steps before and after his death, even if he refused to tell her anything. First, Cathy needed to realize that she, as any wife, had a right to information about her present and future finances. Second, Cathy, as any wife, needed to realize she had to take responsibility to make preparations for herself if nobody else was going to do it. Complaining that her husband wouldn't tell her anything and then doing nothing about it was not a wise option. Having no money for a lawyer, Cathy could have created an Understanding with herself to get as much information as she could from free sources. She could have searched for information about bank accounts, insurance, and other important details. If she had had more money, she could have hired an attorney, an accountant, or other investigators to help gather the information to which she had legal rights. Then, she could have created a plan for her future.

Rather than just yelling at Craig, her discussions could have started, "Craig, I know you don't like to talk about our money; however, I'm really concerned about what I'll do in the future. I don't know how I'll live once you're gone." Because this was an abusive relationship, Craig likely would have said something like, "Well, it's none of your business. I don't want to talk about it. Just leave me alone!" Although this discussion may seem like a waste of time given the circumstances, if Craig had been approached in a noncritical and noncombative way, the outcome might have been different. If approached in a neutral manner, he might not have felt attacked and may have been more forthcoming with the information—he may even have been willing to tell Cathy they had nothing. And if the outcome had not been different, at least Cathy would have known she had taken a stand for herself.

If it weren't an abusive relationship, I would have recommended pursuing it further with Craig. For instance, she could have said, "I know you don't want to talk about it; however, it's really important to me. I know you want me to understand how to take care of myself, and I need information to do it. If you tell me where to find the information, I can look through it, and you don't even need to help me if you don't feel up to it." Or, "I know you don't want to talk about it. However, if you write down a list of what we have, I can go find these things. After that, I won't have to bother you."

Perfectionism

A very private fine line is that between being perfect and being human. I've been known to be a perfectionist. And, of course, that applied to protecting and taking care of my husband. I had to face my humanness and inability to be perfect many times. For instance, one of my husband's lesser falls resulted from stepping on a cat toy that I thought I should have seen and picked up.

Jean, also a perfectionist, took over all the business responsibilities when Joe became ill. When he got to the point of needing a feeding tube in his stomach, she fulfilled that responsibility during her off-work hours. She guiltily admitted to multitasking while she fed him—often balancing the phone on her shoulder to make business calls while feeding him through the tube. A discussion could have begun, "Joe, I'm willing to help with the feeding tube. However, the only way I'll have time to do that is to return phone calls at the same time. Do you mind?" This question would have avoided a one-sided Understanding. Also, if she had asked Joe, the response might have been that it was fine, leaving her with no guilt about multitasking. Or Joe might have responded that they'd get someone else to help out, because she was already overburdened. She couldn't be perfect, didn't have to do it all, or do it all "right." No wife does.

The same applies to others' behaviors. There are going to be accidents, spills, forgotten things, neglected things, broken things, and things simply done wrong by us, friends, our husbands, family, and caregivers. That is the human part. If we expect it, we'll be less devastated when it happens. However, even though it is to be expected, you shouldn't ignore these incidents. When health and safety are at issue, something needs to be said. Such discussions with an employee might begin, "I realize you have a lot of patients to care for and your job is very difficult; however, my husband's safety and comfort is our primary concern. Is there a way I can get you more help so this doesn't happen again?" Or, "Let's figure out a way to prevent this from happening." If it is a family member, often that conversation is more tricky. Jumping to a social and familial issue for a moment, if a person realizes their error and says something, obviously taking responsibility for it, a comment can be made to acknowledge that while trying to make the person feel better: "I realize you spilled the pills all over; however, you didn't do it on purpose, and I'm sure you won't do it again." However, if the person fails to recognize or excuses some repeated thoughtless or dangerous behavior, something stronger may need to be said. The process still is the same, using an "I realize; however…" statement: "Carla, I realize you aren't used to feeding your brother; however, it's really important that you test his soup first to be sure it's the right temperature. Even though I've mentioned that to you before, you keep burning him. I'm sure you don't want to hurt him; however, I'm afraid I'm going to have someone else feed him if this continues."

We may be afraid we'll hurt other people's feelings by pointing out their mistakes. Feelings may get hurt, but the person will survive. Remember, however, if you present your comments in a compassionate way, using the "I realize; however..." statements, it is the listener's choice as to whether or not they wish to feel hurt. Some people, because of their insecurities, will feel hurt by anything we say — and that is their responsibility. Particularly when it comes to safety issues, our husbands' well-being is far more important than worrying about somebody's hurt feelings.

Another being perfect versus being human issue involves wives who haven't been concerning themselves with duties their husband performed, claiming their lack of expertise and avoiding that work. Certainly nothing is wrong with this choice. However, while our husbands are in the process of dying/decline, *somebody* has to take responsibility for the day-to-day operation of the house, or we will have even more problems to face. As I said in the Introduction, "I'm learning far more than I ever cared to." That learning ran quite the gamut. And the list continued to grow over time, even after my husband's death. My opinion is that if we are too overwhelmed to learn about such things, we need to find someone to take over these tasks. Some practicalities simply can't be ignored without problems resulting. Knowing something about these tasks will be beneficial. First, even if you know people to hire, they aren't always available. Second, it is important to know whether the people you are paying to do things are handling them correctly or even at all.

When jobs that were done by your husband are now left completely undone, you can do what Jean did and have your husband teach you how to do them. Jean learned how to cope with and to fix many household problems by getting Joe out of bed and wheeling him to where she needed instruction. Interestingly, it created another level of intimacy for them in the process.

Making Plans

Plans versus no plans can be a very frustrating fine-line issue. Whatever plans existed for the future are ripped away, leaving us feeling cheated. The other side of this is well expressed in Susan's comment, shared earlier, in which she wondered how long a terminal condition really could last. In my situation, I wasn't expecting five or ten years. Along with feeling cheated, Susan also felt stymied, because she couldn't make any plans for her future with such uncertainty in her home.

Remember, all the women in this book were in situations where their husbands were ill for many years, from five to more than twelve. These were not situations where they endured illness for a year or so and then were free to move on to the next phases of their lives. It wasn't that they wanted their husbands dead—they just wanted to be able to create their futures or know when that time might start. As we go through these difficult years, at times it seems as though our past, present, and future have all been taken from us.

At the beginning, most of us put our lives on hold. It is an automatic response, as time and attention have to go to medical appointments and treatments, leaving little time for activities outside basic work and familial duties. We may think we'll be a caregiver for a short time, either because our husbands will get well or they will pass on. Yet a fine-line issue develops over time as it becomes evident that they will not recover and that dying/decline will be an exceedingly slow process for them. For Jean, as the years of Parkinson's went by, she found that all of Joe's and her plans were ruined, that all their retirement plans were scrapped, and that she had missed her chance for the lovely sunset years. Yes, the husband tragically misses these things too, but the focus of this book is the wife. Cathy, Tina, and Mary also were of retirement age, and all of them watched their plans disappear, leaving them with sadness and anger. Now what were they to do? How long would their husbands stay alive? Would they be in nursing homes? Just what would happen? Could they plan? Was it wrong to plan? If they could plan, what would they plan? How could they plan around an unknown?

If you decide you can't go on in limbo like this, it is time for a discussion. The first discussion is with yourself as you go through the preparations needed to form Understandings. Take time to figure out what you want to do at this point in your life. If your husband were well, what activities would you want to do with him? Could you still do some portion of them? Take travel as a simple example. Perhaps your plan was to see the Grand Canyon. Instead of white-water rafting, taking a bus or train tour would work. If travel is out of the question, then perhaps you could go to an IMAX theater nearby that is showing a Grand Canyon movie. If that is out of the question, viewing a DVD about the Grand Canyon at home may be the answer. Perhaps your husband would be open to your going without him and returning home to share videos of your trip. Some semblance of the original plan may still work. Be creative, and keep your eyes open to possibilities.

With Mark and Mary, the discussion began, "Mark, I'm really concerned about what we're going to do during the time you have left. We planned so many nice trips. Do you think we can start going on some right away while you're still feeling pretty good?" Mark was very much in favor of that. He also told Mary that once he was gone, he wanted her to continue doing these things and to see the places they had wanted to go to together — to do it for him. In fact, he wanted her to sprinkle his ashes at several different locations.

Another thing you need to ask yourself is what you, as an individual, wanted to be doing at this time in your life. Did you want to be involved in a sport, take a class, read more, work?

Whatever that desire may be, what portion of it can you do now? If your husband had already passed on, what is it you would want to be doing? Perhaps it would involve the same list of possibilities just mentioned. What portion of that list could you do now, under your current circumstances, if you decided to do so? After thinking through these things, you'll be ready for a discussion.

Tina was very interested in staying fit. Taking care of Tom took up a great deal of her time, and he never liked her to be away from him. Her discussion started, "Tom, I realize you want me here all the time; however, I need to be able to go to exercise class, to take walks, and to go swimming. I've stayed with you as much as I can; however, exercise is very important to me. I'm arranging to do my classes during the times you usually sleep. However, one of the classes doesn't fit your sleep schedule. I'll have someone here with you during that time." Tom wasn't pleased. Tina, knowing that Tom was perfectly safe with the arrangements she made, attended the classes she wanted. Each time he complained, her response was pretty much the same: "I realize you want me to stay home. However, I need to be out for my exercise." Although it is our job to make sure our husbands are safe, it is not our job to make our husbands happy. Only they can do that.

Jean wanted to improve her French. To accomplish that, her plan was to live part of the year with her husband in France, but that plan was ripped away. Not knowing how long her husband would survive, she couldn't make a plan for herself to live there, either. Because she had taken over Joe's role at work along with a lot of the home care, her schedule didn't allow her even to consider adding a French class. Instead, she bought French lessons on DVDs and CDs to use on her computer and to play in her car. In addition, she watched a French television channel to sharpen her skills. Although she couldn't follow her original plan while her husband was alive, she now spends part of each year in France. She lives in a farmhouse she remodeled using skills she learned from her husband.

Susan, Fran, and I, on the other hand, faced our husbands' dying/declines before we were ready for retirement. Initially Susan put her life on hold to be home for her husband any time he was awake. As months of that went by, she felt nothing good came of it. Instead she felt that if she pursued a normal life, that might be more helpful to him. Since Sam spent a great deal of time sleeping and didn't need care at those times, Susan started a business that made her feel alive again. Susan and the others took time to take care of themselves physically, emotionally, and spiritually, which you'll learn about in Chapter 8. These activities were part of how they took themselves out of limbo as they created and executed short-term plans. Fran, rather than leaving her job to take care of Frank, firmly held on to it. She knew she'd need it once Frank passed on. Although my private practice was dissolved due to the time I had to spend away for my husband's cancer care and heart transplant, I later created other business projects I could engage in from home. Some of these entailed short-term plans that could be greatly expanded in the future. I kept my therapy license current in case I wanted to return to the practice later. I put several possibilities in place even though I couldn't give them a time frame or other specifics. And I worked on the parts of the plans I could accomplish within the realities and confines of my husband's many illnesses.

Moving into Reality

The stage of our husbands' illness may determine how we walk the practical fine line between being a cheerleader (advocate) and a realist. If you've been to medical appointments with your husband, you probably have a clear idea of the gloomy, and often thoughtless, way information is presented to him. Two recent visits I've had for minor skin irritations resulted in both doctors beginning their conversations, "Oh yes, we'd better check, because melanoma is quite common in that area." Neither doctor had even begun the exam—yet their first comment threw trauma directly in my face. The moment they actually saw the spots, they declared they were nothing to worry about. But this all-too-common toxic conversation inflicts real damage, and it needs to be counteracted. As the cheerleader (advocate), we can help when our husbands can't do this for themselves. Through the years of my husband's illnesses, I focused a great deal of attention on these issues. Particularly during chemotherapy, I worked directly with doctors and nurses regarding what they should and shouldn't say to and around him during treatments. I even convinced several surgeons to allow a special stuffed toy cat in the operating room with him during his many surgeries. I told my husband when I thought the doctors were wrong with their grim predictions (statistics are about groups and not individuals), supported him when he thought the doctors and labs were wrong (as both sometimes were), and yet never displayed false optimism. If I couldn't agree or give encouragement, I kept quiet.

However, when I saw him showing symptoms of the end drawing near, which occurred in his sleep, I told him what I saw and suggested he do things he needed to do while he still could. I didn't want him to miss opportunities to see or talk to friends one last time. I moved from the cheerleader (advocate) to the realist side, but I did so with compassion—and reluctance. At that point, I felt it was more authentic to be the realist. Authenticity should be your test.

Some of the difficulty with this line is that the realist side can leave us feeling like the "bad guy" in our role as messenger. Part of walking the line is determining whether the message is necessary and if delivering it really is our business. It isn't showing compassion to express a reality for no helpful reason. For instance, it would have been cruel for me to point out to my husband that I saw the signs of his death coming, just so he'd know. It was only when I guessed that he wasn't aware of the signs—and because I knew he wanted to see and to talk to certain people before he died—that I told him.

Susan is an optimist by nature, and Sam was not. A great deal of her energy was spent bolstering him, giving him encouragement, and giving him ideas for how his life could be better. She was so much into the cheerleader mode that she would give information and explain, beg, cry, nag, and even insult him into action—but none of it worked. Good solutions were right there, but he wouldn't take them. He would do things his way but complain anyway. She moved to the realist side by presenting the information and then letting it go. He would use it, or he would not use it—but her job was done. She knew, at some level, that these things weren't her business, yet felt it better to have the information available for Sam in case something might catch his attention.

Of course, on either side of this line, the "I realize; however…" statements can be used. With Jean on the cheerleader side, she could have said to Joe, "I realize this exercise is hard for you to do; however, you know how glad you were the last time you did it." On the realist side, Fran might have said, "Frank, I realize it's very difficult for you to have that talk with your brother; however, you might be running out of time to do it."

Recognizing there are times when it may be none of our business to be the realist with our husbands, it is very important to be one with ourselves. It is easy to get lulled into the cheerleader side, which is the area of hopeful denial described earlier. Although that mode can get us through difficult times by letting us disconnect from them, it can create difficulties down the line when reality cannot be avoided. No matter what terrible and complete physical breakdowns Cathy saw her husband experience, to the very end, she believed he would get well. When he passed on, her grief hit her full force, as she could no longer avoid reality. On the other side of that, women who are hoping their husbands' pain and suffering will end, thus freeing them to move on, need to be realistic in that it may be a long time before that happens.

chapter 7

Social and Familial Issues

S OCIAL AND FAMILIAL ISSUES involve all the other people in our lives: children, relatives, friends, neighbors, clergy, doctors, and helpers. As I discussed earlier, the dilemma of "my way versus his way" underlies all our issues. Although we've created *our* way of functioning in many areas of our marriages, we also know those routines are often thrown out the window when we learn our husbands are terminally ill. Particularly at the beginning, we fall into that protecting-mother mode and create many one-sided Understandings: "I know what you think, want, and need, and I will be in charge of those things. I know what's good and bad for you, so I will make those choices for you. You don't have to do a thing. I will take care of everything." But these one-sided Understandings run on a collision course with frustration and problems in the social and familial areas, where we're dealing with not only his way but also *their* way. Things become much more complicated when we add all those other people's needs and opinions to the mix. Furthermore, *their* way often collides with whatever forms of *our* way we and our husbands have managed to establish during these challenging times.

Being somewhat private people, and of like mind on many issues, my husband and I often said that the whole situation would have been much easier if we had only had to deal with ourselves. Other couples, however, thrive on the inclusion of more family and friends and find that their involvement makes the situation easier for them. Either way, difficult times certainly lie ahead, including many problems in this social and familial area. I'll teach you ways to smooth out those times and to manage or solve the problems.

Whose Business Is It, Anyway?

I'm going to assume that by the time you're reading this book, most family and friends know that your husband is terminally ill. In some families, the relationships may be close, but others may be strained. Either situation may bring surprising twists to this phase. This can be a daunting time, because our children, no matter their ages, are facing the loss of their father. Adult children, in particular, may have the need and feel they have the right to know everything that is going on. This attitude is to be expected and respected but not necessarily acted upon. Somebody else's need does not translate to being our husbands' or our needs. Ultimately, as I said earlier, it is our husbands' disease and their right to decide the course they and it will take. Although social and familial circumstances are not as straightforward as treatment and self-care issues, this approach also applies to decisions regarding who is to be told what.

It is really important to use your communication tools here. At the very least, you need to talk with your husband about the situation. Perhaps both of you think nothing should be held back from anybody, and that choice certainly could simplify things… or not. Perhaps certain types of information can be freely shared but not others. Or you may decide that certain things should be withheld from your children, depending on their ages or perceived ability to handle it. Maybe you'll decide that good news is to be shared regularly, but bad news isn't. You have many options, and they will change over time.

In addition to our children, our husbands' siblings, other relatives, and friends come into play regarding who should be told what and when. Although your decisions about this likely will be modified over time, it is good to start with a framework so you and your husband are on the same page. In whatever format, you should create Understandings, whether written or just verbal. Doing this will be time well spent. I recommend that these Understandings include reviews from time to time as the conditions and circumstances change. You wouldn't want to be operating from a mutual decision that your husband later changes without telling you.

If you are not on the same page as your husband, things can become extremely complicated or troublesome very quickly. Here is one example: Jean became very distressed when Joe started exhibiting more pronounced Parkinson's symptoms. A frequent customer of their business saw the concerned look on her face and asked what was wrong. Jean told her. Later, the customer returned and told Joe how sorry she was to learn he was getting worse. Joe was very upset with Jean, because he didn't want their personal life spilling over into their work life, nor did he like hearing that anyone thought he was getting worse.

Tina and Tom frequently ate at the same restaurant. Because of his bladder-control issues and difficulty walking, Tina asked for tables that were an easy walk to the restroom. One time they went to dinner with his children, who complained about the table location. Tina told them, "We need to be near the restroom in case your father has an 'accident.' He doesn't have good bladder control anymore." Tom was mortified that she shared such a private detail about his decline.

More often, the problem lies in having agreed upon something we think will work but later find it doesn't. Frank didn't want his children to know how much he was deteriorating. Perhaps he didn't want them to worry, or he just was embarrassed that he couldn't function as he had before. Fran agreed not to tell. However, Fran needed help caring for Frank and doing the many things he used to do, and their children were willing to help. Because Frank didn't want the kids to know how badly he was doing, Fran had to fend for herself. Fortunately, Fran and Frank came to a revised Understanding fairly quickly so she could take advantage of the offers of help.

As an extreme example, the husband may decide he doesn't want anyone to be given details about his condition, and yet the wife has been told he just has a few days or weeks to live. He doesn't want his children, siblings, friends, or anyone for that matter to know that information. It may be because he wants them to remember him as he was, he doesn't want to see or to hear from any of these people due to strained relations, or he doesn't have the energy to deal with other people's grief. He may not give a reason, or even fully know why himself. He just doesn't want anyone to be told. I believe that's his right.

Perhaps you would strongly disagree if your husband made that decision, regardless of whether or not you thought he had the right to make it. Assuming your husband is still of sound mind, you then need to have another discussion that ideally would lead to a workable Understanding for both of you. If you cannot reach the Understanding you want and simply agree to disagree, you have a moral decision to make regarding whether or not you'll respect his wishes. Because this action or inaction lies with you, unlike many of the medical decisions, you are in a unique position to easily go against his wishes. You can very likely recall a movie or TV show that depicted a dramatic and wonderful deathbed reconciliation with family or friends that was arranged against the dying person's wishes. This type of scenario may pull at you very strongly and deeply.

Regardless of whether we agree with our husbands' decisions or not, a different problem may arise when we honor those decisions. Suppose you've promised not to tell anyone about his imminent demise, so without any warning to others, your husband passes. When people find out, they feel hurt and angry that they weren't forewarned. Although all those feelings are part of their grief and really aimed toward your husband, they get directed toward you because he's not here. This kind of situation can be a very difficult to handle on top of our own grieving.

Everyone Has an Opinion

When I counsel people who have just learned they have cancer or another life-threatening condition, I suggest they tell very few people. That's because the first reaction from others is usually to tell about their own cancer and how they handled it or to talk about someone they know who had the exact same kind of cancer and what they did or didn't do about it. Finally, they load up the newly diagnosed person with advice on how to do and handle everything, along with a lot of horror stories pertaining to that particular malady. It is no different when we talk about our husbands' terminal illness. Others will tell us how to prevent the death and why or why not the death will happen. Over the years of the dying/decline, the focus will change to how they and their friends had to care for their husbands, how we should get help, whether we should get help, which people to hire, and the ins and outs and horror stories pertaining to each step of the way. Eventually, the input, advice, opinions, and horror stories will center around end-of-life issues, funerals, and what to do after our husbands pass. The point is, the input from others isn't going to end, and we need ways to handle it. If you don't mind that input, you have no coping techniques to learn. But for many people enduring this stress, the last thing they need is an unwelcome barrage of advice. If a person wants to share his or her stories and opinions and you don't want to hear them, you have several ways to handle that situation.

Anita, one of Tina's friends, found out that Tom was on Antabuse, which causes a person to vomit if they ingest any alcohol. She said to Tina, "I really think it's cruel to give Antabuse to Tom." Tina had many options for responses, such as: "Thank you for sharing that. I appreciate your concern"; or "I realize you really think it's cruel to give Antabuse to Tom; however, we've decided to use it"; or "I realize you really think it's cruel to give Antabuse to Tom; however, I'm not comfortable discussing private matters." Tina didn't have to make Anita "wrong" for Tina to be "right." And she had no obligation to discuss this decision with Anita just because Anita felt it was important. This very simple method, repeated over and over again, can be used to respond to any of those unwelcome opinions or pieces of information.

Ultimately, if Anita had a strong opinion, Tina could have suggested that Anita should mention this directly to Tom by saying something such as: "I realize you really think it's cruel to give Antabuse to Tom; however, you'll have to take that up with him, because it was his decision." Of course, if Anita had decided to act on it, it would have brought up the issue of visitors, which I discuss next.

The Hottest Button

One of the most difficult social and familial issues occurs when, even after an Understanding has been created, our husbands make a sudden switch to the ideas or opinions that other family members or friends present. That change often occurs without our husbands consulting or including us. This can be particularly annoying and humiliating if your husband agrees with others on an issue about which you have been trying to change his mind or behavior. For instance, you've talked, pleaded, and done everything you could think of to get your husband to stop smoking, to try a certain treatment, or to switch to a certain doctor. He has refused time and time again. Then, a friend of his visits, and he suddenly agrees to do it...all within the course of a half hour. Cathy had this kind of incident happen on many occasions, and it really irked her. It seemed Craig thought that what anybody else said had more value, so he would go along with it. It was not uncommon for him to change from suggestion to suggestion to suggestion, even going back to a previous idea when a friend came along and gave him the original idea—the one that was Cathy's.

Jean and Joe had been very pleased with his endocrinologist, and Joe seemed to be feeling better following her protocol. Then Joe's sister came to visit. She didn't think Joe was doing all that well. Her neighbor had gone to a different doctor and didn't have symptoms like Joe's anymore. Joe's sister thought this new doctor was the best one ever, so after meeting with his domineering sister, Joe decided to switch to the new doctor. Jean was livid.

Although it didn't happen, Anita could have spoken with Tom or his children about the Antabuse, causing him to stop taking it. These things happen...a lot.

Even when the switch is to an outcome we desire, it may be difficult for us to accept. Jean had been giving her all to make sure Joe was fine. She spent countless hours with him, went to many doctor's appointments, administered many of his medications, and knew his condition inside and out. Jean's issues weren't just that Joe changed his mind so easily, but that it represented a lack of respect for her and her opinions. It broke an Understanding when he created a one-sided one and devalued Jean, along with her constant care and effort. Those elements constitute the most difficult aspect of social and familial issues. This is, by far, the single biggest issue wives reported regarding friends and family.

Susan felt a similar devaluing when Sam would get dressed up for visitors but not for her. This appearance also gave visitors the illusion that things were better in the house than they were. As a result, concerns she shared with friends were invalidated when the visitor told her how great Sam looked.

About all we can do when it is a medical decision, unless we have medical power of attorney, is try to create Understandings about how such incidents can be handled in the future, and then do our anger work, as described in Chapter 5, "Comprehending Our Emotions: Life in the Guilt Factory."

When Someone Asks

Even though families and social groups may know that death is looming, only those living in our homes really know what's going on with our husbands' illness and the dynamics surrounding it. We aren't likely to share details, particularly the ones dealing with intimate caregiving. Most of the time when people ask how our husbands are doing, they're just being polite and are looking for simple answers without specifics. After all, almost everyone has something difficult going on in their lives and doesn't really want to get involved in our problems as well. You may feel that's a relief, particularly after several years, because you've found, unfortunately, that the questioning often implies judgment. On the other hand, you may be offended to know that many people really don't care.

I caution wives to be sensitive about unloading their woes when someone inquires. If you tell all, people will stop asking and may go out of their way to avoid you. None of the ladies I interviewed had that happen. But I think you know those people who, when you politely ask them how they are, tell you everything…and you end up feeling sorry you asked.

So how should you handle it when you don't want to share, only want to share a certain amount, or only want to share with certain people? Some women find they isolate themselves in order to avoid the onslaught of questions and barrage of information. This response isn't healthy or necessary.

I recommend using the communication tools described earlier, along with creating rote responses. It will be helpful to have several set responses ready when someone asks how your husband is doing. Fran made up and practiced some of her responses, later revising and adding to them after she found what worked. "Thank you for asking—he's doing as well as can be expected," she'd say. Or, "Frank is busy with treatments and rests a lot in between," and "Frank is handling this well now, and I'll let him know you asked about him." Notice that this last example not only gives a response, without giving detail, but also allows a conversation to end. It is a gentle way to stop the conversation while acknowledging the person's concern. Ironically, friends may not be comfortable asking and therefore may be glad you did this.

You will, however, encounter exceedingly nosy people. If someone pursues questioning about your husband, your "I realize; however…" statements can be powerful tools: "I realize you want to know how Frank is; however, I'd rather talk about something else right now"; "I realize you want to know how Frank is; however, this really isn't a good time for me"; or "I realize you want to know how Frank is; however, I'm really not comfortable talking about it." Fran used this one, particularly when she felt that talking about it might bring her to tears, taking all her energy to hold herself together.

When your children or close family members ask, you probably will give longer responses. These people are most apt to push the questioning because of their extreme and genuine concern and perceived right to know. These same tools may be used with them, although these people may be more sensitive to responses they might consider dismissive. Remember, however, you are acting from the Understanding that you and your husband created, and you are honoring his wishes. To prevent sensitivity issues, it may be wise to share that Understanding with your children and family members so they know what to expect.

You may only need to revert to these seemingly mechanical methods if the questioning goes too far. Nothing about these responses needs to be impolite or unkind, no matter the behavior of the person asking. You can use these tools as a good framework on which to build your answers. When using the "I realize; however…" statements, remember to start with the exact wording the other person used.

For instance, your son asks how Dad's blood work came out. It wasn't very good, and you've decided only to give positive information. Your response may be, "I realize you want to know how Dad's blood work came out; however, we want to wait for another test to be done before we discuss it with anyone." Or you may want to loosen up the wording a bit but still withhold information, saying, "Joe, I'm sure it's difficult for you not knowing all the details about Dad; however, Dad and I agreed we would only share certain information. We'll tell you as much as we can, but I can't share this right now." Or it may be, "Dad doesn't want me discussing that with you right now. I'll let you know when he tells me it's all right to share it."

Public Face with Private Pain

Although we may tire of endlessly being asked how our husbands are doing, at times we also like to be remembered and shown concern by our friends. Susan had a rote response when friends asked about Sam. She'd say, "He's doing well. And I'm fine, too!" This answer made the point that she, too, was going through something—it wasn't just Sam. When she talked with people, she didn't want them to feel sorry for her, but she wanted them to understand. And if we keep a lot of information private, most people will have no idea how bad it might be behind our closed doors. We put on our happy faces as much as we can, and we do it for a number of reasons. We don't want to burden others, we don't want to prompt questioning, and we are trying to keep things as normal as possible. Susan was in such private pain that it seemed to her that "real life ha[d] become a dirty little secret." However, once people knew of Sam's illness and it was no longer a completely private matter, she preferred that people ask her what was going on rather than having them make up something and spread rumors.

Another element of the divide between our public faces and private pain involves the way we treat our husbands in public. Sometimes, because we want others to understand and to empathize with us, we may have a tendency to pick on our husbands when we have an audience. We let our private pain bleed through when we are in public. It seems that if we draw others' attention to our husbands' faults, friends will reinforce our feelings about them. However, the more likely outcome is that people will not understand our motivations and will feel sorry for our husbands and think less of us.

Some things should remain private. One of those is criticism of our husbands. I'm not suggesting that you should be critical of your husband in private, either, but you are human and stressed, and sometimes it just comes out.

Mary was very concerned about Mark's appearance. Mark lost a lot of weight, and his Parkinson's caused his posture to deteriorate. Because of this condition, it didn't look like Mark was dressed properly. Mary was concerned that others might think she was failing in her wifely duties. So, she commented to him, in front of others, that he looked like he was slouching in his suit. Mark and everyone else involved were deeply embarrassed for both of them. Mary later made an Understanding with herself to stop this behavior.

Jean admitted that when her neighbor came over so she could have an evening out or a good night's sleep, she complained about Joe's behavior in front of him. Sometimes she'd say, "You'd better be careful, because Joe isn't going to remember to clean himself," but with a tone that was critical rather than informative. She regretted having done that and later apologized to Joe.

In cases such as this, it is wise to reflect on the passage shared earlier and consider whether what you say will improve upon the silence. Since it may not be easy to remember to do that, it might be a good idea to make a little sign with this phrase and post it several places around the house. It will be a reminder not only to you but to your husband and to anyone else who may come into your home:

> *Before you speak,*
> *ask yourself,*
> *is it kind,*
> *is it necessary,*
> *is it true,*
> *does it improve on the silence?*

The contrast between public face and private pain also encompasses a profound change in our social lives. Suddenly we are excluded, or have to exclude ourselves, from the very events and activities that could make our lives more pleasant—little, happy, often pretty diversions, the joyful connections with family and friends that could nurture and heal.

Although you may wish to have a normal social life, including your husband in it, you may find that his illness makes it less likely for people to invite you places or to accept your invitations. It may be that others are afraid something will happen to him while he is in their homes or that a great deal of accommodation needs to be made because of his illness, whether that is completely changing a meal plan, arranging special seating, or finding a way to get him into and out of a house. Grandpa doesn't get invited to visit as often, because he's spilled things, soiled himself, or acted up at the dinner table. Sam doesn't get invited, because he's never clean. Mark doesn't get invited, because he might fall. Joe doesn't get invited, because he needs a feeding tube.

And you may turn down invitations for many of the same reasons. Because my husband needed so much dialysis, travel to visit his family became almost impossible. When absolutely necessary, like after a hurricane, arrangements could be made in another city to continue dialysis, but it would still have meant he'd be sleeping most of the time. Air travel was not good for him, either, and that caused him to miss his son's out-of-state wedding.

People may not want to come to your home because it holds too many physical reminders of how much your husband is declining. Your home may not be pleasant anymore, and your husband simply may not have the energy to be involved socially.

Although some social and familial connections may cause you great stress, you'll see more fully in the next chapter how important certain ones can be to help sustain you during these difficult times.

A change in our identity creates another aspect of our public face and private pain struggles. A split develops between our normal identity and our husband-is-dying identity. Our husbands may change their identity from that of "strong, healthy man" to "dying man." Understandably, this role shift may be difficult for them to handle, but this has an impact on us as wives as well. People think of Susan as "you know, the one whose husband is dying," rather than as "the one who works at city hall." In a sense, we are caught up in the same wave and are looked at or treated differently because of it. You may like it when that happens, as being a recognized martyr gives you a sense of purpose and importance. But if you are bothered by it, you will find it is even more important to stay involved with family and friends doing customary activities. This way, they will think of you as "Tina…

the one who goes to my church" or "Fran…the teacher." Maintaining our normal identities helps keep us grounded and helps prevent a sick life from becoming our new norm.

For many, it is hard to balance having a normal life with the sick life because of the pulls this sick life has on them. For years and years and years, it is at the forefront of almost everything we do and every decision we make. This is a big part of our private pain. We'd much rather be doing enjoyable things with our husbands, not helping them get dressed or giving them medicine. We'd much rather be making decisions about the next vacation we'll take with our husbands, not figuring out what we'll do when they can no longer feed themselves. This pain stays private because of how others would react if we said anything.

My husband was on an extremely low-sodium diet for many years, so I made a special version of pizza. I remember several people asking what would be the first thing I would do after my husband died. I said I wanted to just sit down on the sofa, watch TV, and eat some good pizza. This, to me, would signal the end of the sick life and the return to normal life. It was very simple and probably sounded silly, but it was very profound. It was more than a month after he died before I was able to bring myself to do it.

Visitors and Privacy

Because our husbands may be ill for a long time, the issue of visitors will come up many times. You may love having visitors, because it gives you a break. On the other hand, those visitors may create more work for you if they expect you to entertain them while your husband is asleep, to shop and prepare meals for them, or to clean up after them. You probably already have more complicated preparation and cleaning demands due to changing dietary, sanitary, and medication needs and the schedules related to them.

Outsiders coming into the house can greatly complicate and throw off our rhythms. This can result in missed meds, inappropriate food, and sanitary accidents. Often we may have special medical equipment in the house, whether it is something as simple as a cane or a walker or as elaborate as special toilets, wheelchairs, beds, IVs, or other devices. It is not as easy to move around our homes, and things are more crowded than they were before. On top of that, our husbands may have an episode, get sick, fall, or have a sanitary accident while a visitor is there. An outsider's presence could make it harder or easier for us, depending on who is there and if the person is capable of and willing to help. Even if we love having visitors, it is just not always an easy matter.

If you have younger children at home, it may be wise to look at what having visitors does to their routines. Most likely, their father's illness has already greatly affected their normal routines, even though you've tried to maintain normal-life structures for the sake of everyone's sanity. Depending on what the visitors want to do and when they want to come, they can be a help or hindrance. Over time, you'll start to figure out which it is, and for which people.

Just as children and friends have a need and feel a right to have information about our husbands, they have a need and feel they have a right to visit. Once again, their desires are to be expected and respected, but not necessarily acted upon. Somebody else's need does not translate into being our husbands or our needs. Again, your husband's wishes should prevail in terms of whom he will or will not see. Because you usually are directly affected by the visits, your needs and wishes also need to be included in how to handle them.

So how should you handle this kind of situation? Once again, it is time for a conversation with your husband. You may be thinking this whole approach to caregiving sure requires a lot of talking. Yes, it does. But if you object to talking it through, you will soon realize this may be a talk-now-or-get-annoyed-and-argue-later scenario. The more of these issues you resolve ahead of time, the more easily things will flow. You won't be able to figure out everything ahead of time, and exceptions will always be made, but having a basic framework in place will be very helpful.

You need to decide what will work for you, and you need to realize that what's appropriate likely will change over time. You may decide that certain people may drop in unannounced or that everyone must call first. Or you may decide that Sunday is family day and nobody outside the family is to come that day, unless someone is passing through town and this is the only day they can visit and you therefore need to make an exception.

You may decide that no visitors are to come during medication times, mealtimes, or treatment times — just like in a hospital. The hospital model is a good one, because the staff understand well how much more difficult it is to accomplish things with extra people underfoot, so they do something about it.

Jean and Joe's children lived far away, so they weren't able to visit on a regular basis. As we have learned, Jean had Joe teach her how to repair things in the house, so she became the handyperson and was in charge of maintenance. When the kids visited, they weren't used to that and tended to bypass Jean, causing more problems. They'd go to their dad, asking him what to do about the garbage disposal and discounting or ignoring Jean's new role and abilities. Then she had to deal with them in addition to fixing the garbage disposal, making her life even more stressful. Jean needed to do something about this situation.

On the other hand, Cathy welcomed the help of visitors. She often heard them offer to help, but, ironically, Craig would turn them down. She shared, "I'm so angry when others offer to help him and he pretends he's so strong and doesn't need their help." Of course, if he then turned to Cathy for help, she had the option to decline. Certainly they needed to have a discussion about this type of behavior so they could have come to an Understanding. If he wouldn't discuss it, which was common for Craig, she could have told him that she would comply with his request this one time, but if he were to turn down help for this issue in the future, she would not assist him.

You and your husband may have created an Understanding that no visitors are allowed at the time you come home from work. This is not only a transition time for you to switch roles but a very busy time, as you catch up with things for the house and your husband. Yet your husband's pal George drops in time and time again just when you're trying to get dinner ready. Your husband won't say anything to him, because he doesn't want to hurt his feelings, totally ignoring yours. And because you still manage to get dinner ready, it doesn't affect your husband in any way, except that he may hear you complain. After further discussions with your husband, likely using "I realize; however…" statements, it might be appropriate to share with George the Understanding that you and your husband created. That approach is actually respectful of George. Another possibility would be to sit down with George and your husband, enjoy the visit, and delay cooking until George leaves. Your husband may get upset that his meal isn't ready when he wants it, but logical consequences come into play here, and he gets to decide whether your feelings are as important as George's. Are you going to enable this behavior or not?

This brings up another side of this type of issue involving the "Big C" (codependency). Let's say George likes to drop over each day while you're at work. Your husband likes this, but you don't, because you'd prefer that your husband get more rest. George's visits do not require any extra work on your part, and you wouldn't even know he visited if your husband didn't mention it. In this case, it doesn't affect you, so it is not your business. Certainly you can express your concern about your husband's lack of rest, but beyond that, you need to let it go.

The rule of thumb is that I stay out of it if it doesn't affect me. But if it *does* affect me, I have a right to be involved. That doesn't mean I get to have my way, but I do have a right to create an Understanding about it.

One of the most difficult social and familial circumstances I had to deal with involved visits from my husband's children and grandchildren during his last Christmas. All the adults knew he had planned to stop dialysis in the near future, which meant he would only have five to ten days to live after that. Regardless of whether or not he went through with his plan, it still was pretty clear to everyone that this would be his last Christmas. We (my husband and I) decided to make it as special as we could. We took his energy level and schedule, along with the amount of work it would mean for me, into account. At that time, he spent every other day on dialysis, with only one two-day break each week. He slept most of the day and night on the days he didn't go to dialysis. This basically left only one day a week during which he had some energy, albeit limited.

Added to Christmas were his son's birthday on the 26th and his birthday on the 27th, so there were many special events happening all at once. Working closely with my husband, I created a "Children's Christmas" for the grandchildren on Christmas Day, having them arrive a half hour before their parents so they could decorate cookies, thus creating special alone time for my husband with them. Then the adults came, but they were given just a two-hour window for their visit. The next day, a ladies' lunch was scheduled outside the house when my husband was on dialysis. On the 27th, we had a birthday buffet for my husband at the house, but for just two hours. Then a final Christmas dinner/birthday event was held on the 28th at a favorite club. The key to making this happen was not only taking the time to create an Understanding but informing everyone of the plans ahead of time so they knew what to expect.

As discussed previously, quite a discrepancy often exists between how things look to others and what's really going on. Even though everyone knew my husband was considering going off dialysis, his family didn't really have a sense of how awful he felt or how much time he needed to sleep and thus this regimentation didn't make them very happy, although they did go along with it. Even though we had created an Understanding, I became the bad guy, because I was the messenger and the schedule monitor, ensuring what my husband wanted. But the family's feelings and reactions were most understandable. Leaving the final Christmas dinner and birthday event was painful for everyone, knowing that it likely would be the last time they would see their father, and, for most, it was.

Rather than wishing to visit or to be visited by family, our husbands may decide they want to spend many of their last days traveling or doing something unusual. This decision might be something we, our family, and friends may or may not applaud. I recall boarding a ship for a cruise. I looked at one passenger and said to my husband, "That man is dying." He did die on the cruise. I'm assuming he and his wife knew he didn't have long to live. It likely didn't make a pleasant trip for his widow, but she may have known that's what her husband wanted and was pleased that he died on a cruise rather than in a hospital. I hope that his family and friends were supportive as well.

Conversely, our husbands may have dream adventures or activities that would involve many family and friends, so they invite many to share in a final celebration. There is no end to the diverse ways a husband may wish to socialize or to be with family and friends as he faces his demise. Once again, discussions and Understandings will help accomplish what your husband desires.

Ceremonies and Services

In my opinion, the decisions about what will happen to our husbands' bodies and the accompanying ceremonies belong to them. It can be seen as a separate right or an integral part of how they handle their illness. I well understood, probably for the first time, during my husband's funeral that the event was for those of us left behind. I very much appreciated everyone who was there for me and to honor him. That being said, I also believe he had the right to decide how his funeral should be handled or to decide not to have one at all. My husband had a memorial service followed by a burial service for his cremains six months later.

Regardless of whether or not you share my opinion, what happens at this time has the potential to be extremely contentious. Others will have strong opinions that may conflict with yours. Arrangements usually inspire excessive social and familial input and cause pressures that are heightened when grief is added to the mix. The good news is that you can be prepared for it.

Planning for this time is a very important discussion to have with your husband. To keep things simple, the first discussions should just be between your husband and you. Then, depending on what you decide, you may wish to include others in the discussions to create further Understandings. For instance, if you decide you want input or participation (not necessarily the same thing) from children, siblings, friends, clergy, or others, it is wise to include them in the process now so you don't run into problems at the time your husband passes. Similarly, if you decide you want input from some and not others, it is wise to involve those whose help you want now so they have a clear understanding later that the others are not to be included. Even though you're likely overwhelmed with everything else and don't want to deal with the thought of your husband's passing, you'll be very glad you handled this ahead of time.

Of course, this brings up a situation in which you may want to have this discussion and your husband doesn't. It is not totally uncommon for a man to say, "I'll be dead. What do I care?" Go back to Chapter 3, and you'll see what to do about that. The result may be that if your husband doesn't care about what happens when he dies (and if you're not trying to control him, you'll see that's a perfectly acceptable option) or he simply doesn't want to discuss it (again, his choice), you get to decide. And then as you begin making plans, it is wise to have discussions and to create Understandings involving more people, if you choose.

The other side of this issue is the possibility that you don't want to have the discussion about funerals because *you* don't want to face it. This certainly is an option, and you have some reasonable courses of action. As I say in Chapter 3, "If your husband brings up a topic you don't wish to discuss, you may respond, 'I realize you want to talk to me about your funeral plans; however, all I can do at this point is listen.' If the issue is too emotionally charged, another option is to have him give that information to someone you trust and respect, and then have that person discuss it with you." For the funeral topic, in particular, it would be wise to create an Understanding, such as, "Since talking about funeral plans is too difficult for me, we agree to let our daughter, Jessica, be in charge of those plans." Of course, Jessica needs to be included in a discussion and Understanding.

If you do something like that, you need to be careful about putting in your two cents after you've already given the job to somebody else. However, you can include the stipulation in the Understanding that you will review the plans at the time of death to see if you've changed your mind. It is wise to include that type of "out," so the "Jessicas" can anticipate possibly having their jobs taken away later on.

Sam made his wishes quite clear to Susan. He was an atheist and did not want any kind of funeral service or memorial. She felt he had the right to decide what he wanted and had no trouble doing what he asked. The children also were fine having no service, feeling they had all been through enough without enduring a funeral. Interestingly, some of Sam's former friends decided to have a memorial event, thus meeting their own needs while totally ignoring Sam's wishes. As I said relating to the Big

C, "I can stay out of it if it doesn't affect me." Although it may not be easy, we can ignore such things. You might need to do your anger work relating to it, but beyond that, if it doesn't involve you, it is not your business.

Just as my husband and I created an Understanding about the way his funeral would be handled, so did Susan and Sam. Except for Cathy, the same was true for the most of the other ladies in this book. Tina's husband is still alive.

Jean joined the Jewish faith for Joe when they married. This occurred so many years ago that they had little difficulty getting everyone to understand what this would mean when he died. However, this is exactly the type of situation that provides a brewing pot for difficulties and is one for which having explicit Understandings is wise.

Even though Cathy's husband had been ill for many years, and it seemed obvious from what doctors told them that his death was imminent, Cathy and Craig never discussed the possibility of his death. She thought at one point that he knew it was inevitable, but he just never discussed it with her. More than six years later, she said, "I wish he had, but I wish a lot of things — but it is too late now." Not having the communication tools, she never brought it up either. Surprisingly, "One of the main reasons we didn't bring it up," she shared, "was because I knew how much he wanted to beat the cancer, and I tried to always keep him as positive as I could. So if I had even started to talk about it, he would have thought that I didn't think he was going to make it." I found this an interesting gift they gave each other. He most likely knew he would die but was staying positive for her.

All she knew was that he wanted his ashes placed at home plate where he used to play baseball. When he died, he was cremated, and no service took place. In this case, Cathy had no money to pay for any kind of service or burial, so nobody questioned it, and their children had no problem with the way it turned out.

But this topic certainly has the potential for extreme controversy. If you and your husband disagree, then this is one of those circumstances where conversations toward creating an Understanding are critical. And this may also be a time of personal soul-searching as you decide whether or not you will honor his wishes. If you totally disagree with your husband's wishes and he will not change them, you need to decide what your moral obligation is.

Even though you and your husband agree on what will be done, the children and other relatives may want it their way. Part of the Understanding you create with your husband needs to include what to do about the others and a decision regarding whether or not you should bend to their desires. An example that came up for Mary: Her husband had been in the military and wanted to have the American flag presentation as part of the funeral. Their children were very antimilitary and made quite an issue about this. However, Mary made it clear that this presentation was their father's wish and it was going to be included, which it was, without incident. To accomplish this, using the "I realize; however…" statements would be appropriate: "I realize you don't want anything military-related in the funeral; however, your father asked to have it."

I spoke earlier about the gift of time. This is one of those places where we can take full advantage. If your husband is agreeable, you need to have discussions so you don't have to handle this alone when you're grieving the most. This was a gift my husband gave to me.

chapter 8

Self-Care

WE GET REALLY TIRED of being told to take care of ourselves. Do people really think we don't take care of ourselves on purpose? Don't they understand that we would if we could? Who the heck has the time or energy to do it?! And why don't they just mind their own business and stop giving us these *helpful* suggestions, as if this never entered our minds?

We're trying to manage our roller-coaster-ride emotions, figure out how to carry out our new roles and balance them with our old roles, manage the house and children, cope with the changes our husbands' dying has made in the marriage, figure out sex and intimacy in these new circumstances, do all the practical things that still need to be done, and then maybe even get some sleep. Add to that the pressure that friends, family, and society put on us to devote ourselves to our husbands, and we end up feeling that we're doing something bad or inappropriate if we give attention to ourselves.

Books and websites on caregiving offer worthwhile, commonsense advice. We already know a lot of what they suggest: Eat right, get plenty of sleep, exercise, take time for yourself, stay connected with friends, stay spiritually involved, seek therapy if appropriate, etc. Yet we still ignore most of that. Can we really afford to do so? Why should we take care of ourselves, and how can we get ourselves to do it?

Why should we take care of ourselves? That's pretty simple. The example of the oxygen mask on an airplane is a good one. Airline attendents always direct adult passengers to put oxygen masks on themselves *before* helping children or others with theirs. If you aren't well, you won't be able to help your husband. If you're dead, you won't be able to help your husband—dramatic, but true. Some wives think that if they're sick, they'll have a legitimate reason not to help their husbands, and it will be a break for them. Others think that if they get sick, people will see how hard they've been working and give them some attention for a change.

Two of the women I interviewed had been lectured, quite strongly, by their doctors, because they put all their energy into taking care of their husbands and were suffering emotionally and physically from it. They were asked whether they wanted to shorten their lives and told that their health was as important as that of their husbands. They were directed, quite explicitly, to get away from their husbands if it came to a choice between their spouses and themselves. The issue is *that* serious.

In most cases, he's dying and you're not. Although you may think that you won't have reason to live after your husband dies, most women would like to go on with their lives. If you don't take care of yourself during your husband's dying process, you set yourself up for unhealthy and difficult years after he passes. No matter the reason you choose for taking care of yourself—for him, for you, for your kids, for guilt…any reason will do—let's look at how that can be done and how others do it. It might surprise you.

The wives I interviewed did two things so they could take care of themselves. First, they gave themselves permission to do so. Sometimes this was only in small ways and after much struggle over the issue, but, eventually, they decided it was all right. Second, they came up with ways that worked for them, given their finances and freedom. Although these examples may not illustrate the ways you wish to take care of yourself, the ideas presented might spark your imagination.

Tina loves her husband immensely and gives him excellent and loving care, yet she still does an incredible job of taking care of herself. She was born and raised in Argentina. Every year, she visits her family for an entire month. Her time with Tom takes more and more out of her each year, and she finds it harder and harder to keep up her energy. Because she understands the importance of taking care of herself, she told friends and family that if Tom dies while she is away, "Don't call me. Just put him on ice, and I'll take care of it when I come home." And she's serious! To protect her own health, she is willing to risk the uproar this situation could create among family and friends. A very practical woman, she realizes she can neither predict nor control the time of Tom's death. She also believes that her husband will make a decision, on some level, as to whether or not he wishes to die in her company, so this works for her.

Cathy didn't have much money or transportation. Sometimes she took walks in her neighborhood to relax. Primarily, she took "inner" vacations in her living room. Along with using the Boulder Activity to process the anger she felt toward herself and her husband, she chanted, meditated, read, and did affirmations while her husband slept. In essence, she escaped into herself in healthy ways.

Being totally overwhelmed, Cathy didn't care if the house wasn't perfect for visitors. She figured if they thought it was not clean enough, they could pitch in and help. This was particularly true when her children and grandchildren descended on the house, expecting to be entertained and fed. If they didn't bring and prepare food for themselves, they didn't get to eat. She took care of the visitor issue and herself by setting boundaries for what she would and would not do.

Susan liked "shop therapy." This isn't to suggest that you should medicate with shopping or get into debt. Susan, however, could afford it and really liked high-end shopping areas. Although she certainly enjoyed buying nice things for herself and others, the main idea was to get out of the house and into a pretty environment. Many shopping centers are beautiful havens. And regardless of whether or not you have money to spend, you can enjoy a lovely refuge. You can do the same in many houses of worship.

Shop therapy may be as simple as going to a flea market, going to a dollar store, or just buying some new T-shirts at Walmart. Shop therapy helps because it has a forward, positive feel to it, which counters the stuck feeling of your situation. Buying something new also gives the feeling that a future does exist.

Mary took care of herself by staying involved socially. While Mark was living at home, he was able to care for himself long enough for her to have lunch with friends. Although some criticized her for leaving her husband at home and having fun when he couldn't, she did what she needed to do for herself. When Mark moved to a nursing home, Mary regularly visited galleries and museums, along with her other social activities, rather than spending all of her days sitting with him at the caregiving facility. At first she felt guilty about not being with him all the time, but then she realized that if she didn't take care of her social life, she wouldn't have one after he died. Mary simply was preparing for her future.

Fran and Frank had difficulties over sex. Because Frank was

a sex addict, Fran took care of herself by limiting sex to just one night a week, removing a constant pressure while acknowledging her husband's wishes. In addition, Fran had some good friends from where she taught, and she arranged to spend one Saturday a month and one evening a month doing something fun with them. She also took advantage of any breaks in her class schedule to share immediate concerns with her best friends.

Jean, as you saw in the Understanding she created (see page 66), took time for herself one night every week. She arranged for a neighbor to come in to stay with Joe while she went to a jazz club. She also arranged to have someone come one night a week to spend the entire night with Joe so she could take a sleeping pill and get a night of good sleep. Personally, I used to love the nights my husband had to stay in the hospital. Those were the nights I knew he was well cared for and was safe. Then I could turn off my "mother's ears" and sleep in peace.

In some cases, pursuing these activities requires money to hire help, but you might be able to get a friend, a neighbor, or a family member to assist. Don't be afraid to ask. And that brings me back to some basics, because asking for help may stop you in your tracks.

One of the greatest annoyances for many wives, as Cathy expressed, is that their husbands turn down help from friends. Because our husbands may be ill for many years, people may forget about us and not offer help, particularly if we've turned it down in the past. After a while, if we don't ask, help isn't going to just appear.

During one of my husband's hospitalizations, I noticed a surgical nursing assistant named Livingston who seemed very capable. I asked him whether he did private-duty work. He usually didn't, but he agreed to do it for us. As my husband's health declined, I came to rely on Livingston more and more. Be aware of your needs, keep your eyes open, and ask for help.

Something else I did for myself was participate in yoga classes and work with a trainer two times a week. Not only did this get me out of the house doing something healthy, but it allowed me to be in a positive environment. I stayed active in other organizations where I was surrounded by positive friends and uplifting activities. Twice a year, we also arranged to have one of my husband's sons stay with him while I took short trips to see relatives and friends.

Manufacture Time

Because insufficient time is a major deterrent to taking care of yourself, start by creating more of it. In Chapter 5 I explained how codependency creates extra work. Ask yourself these questions: What am I taking on that I really don't need to? What can I get rid of, eliminate, delegate, let my husband do, or insist that my husband do? What jobs can I give away? How much time can I save by eliminating the nagging that never works?

If you're spending time doing anything for your husband that he could do for himself—or things for others that they could do for themselves—particularly if these are things you don't want to do, create time for yourself by not doing them. You can add a lot of time to your days by creating Understandings that if your husband doesn't accept help offered by others, you won't do that work either. It is that simple. Not necessarily easy, but simple.

Here's one way I created more time for myself. Following my husband's heart transplant, people were calling for updates on his progress. It became an enormous chore for me to handle these calls in between runs to the hospital. So I bought an answering machine that allowed callers to select one of three options. The first option allowed them to leave messages. For the second option, I recorded the latest information on my husband's progress. For the third, I left the contact information for the hospital where he was staying. Not only did this save me a lot of work, time, and stress, but most callers were pleased to know they could get this information without disturbing me. Even simple, practical things can save a lot of time and energy.

Stop Energy Drains

Anger and disturbing thoughts not only create negative outcomes but they also steal our energies. You need to pay attention to your thoughts, as they provide useful information. If you're ruminating and continuously mulling over something, you need to notice what that "something" is. It is likely that you need to take some action. Ruminating without taking action just wastes your time and energy. Perhaps it is time to talk your way to an Understanding with someone or with yourself. If the situation is something you can't do anything about, you'll likely feel angry and need to do the Boulder Activity (see page 78). Although it takes a little time to work through that, you'll free up more time and energy as a result. Back off from issues that you won't win and do something else.

Our thoughts create our images, and our images create our actions and outcomes. Although you may not realize it, you do have control over your thoughts. You can be the boss in the Guilt Factory and determine what gets produced there. You can take care of yourself by using thought interruption and thought replacement. The brain works very much like a computer and doesn't pay attention to whether or not what we run through it is true. We run a lot of garbage through our brains/computers that *we* think is true. Start noticing the thoughts you have: If they don't make you feel good, start replacing them with ones that make you feel better, even if you don't believe them. If you continually tell yourself, "I'm so miserable," change it to, "I'm fine. I can make it through this." You don't have to believe a word of it, but your brain will start to act on it. You may even notice an immediate change in your posture when you change your thought.

Always put into your mind what you want to do rather than what you want to avoid, eliminating "not" statements. It isn't that the brain can't process not statements, as some say, but the *way* it processes them causes trouble. If I say, "I'm not going to think of a red car," my brain has to create an image of a red car so it knows what it shouldn't think about. So if you want to think about a green car, tell yourself, "I'm going to think about a green car." That's the reason it is much more effective to caution a child with "walk" rather than "don't run." This approach is very simplistic but very helpful with our computer-like brains.

Depression is said to be suppressed anger. Along with things about which we're happy and grateful, we've got a lot of things that cause anger and depression during this time. After all, our husbands are dying. You may feel waves of depression, which are easy to identify, but you may not recognize other signs. You may find that you lack concentration or are inattentive and pass that off as being tired. You may feel irritable or easily agitated. Although these reactions are to be expected, they could be signs of depression. These are signals to take some action, whether it is doing the Boulder Activity, talking to a friend, or seeking professional help. Although these feelings are normal and to be expected, you'll want to do something about them so they don't escalate.

Holding in any emotion drains your energy and can destroy your health. Allow yourself to experience your full range of emotions. Susan allowed herself to get the worst crying out of her system until she got tired of it. Of course, she shed tears at other times, but she didn't allow her grief to keep draining her energy.

The Delicate Topics —
Love, Sex, Intimacy, and Affairs

As with emotional issues, no value judgments are placed on these "delicate" topics. It is to be expected that medical conditions are going to change our sex lives or the way we think about or approach sex. Your husband may become impotent from his illness or medications or simply no longer have a sex drive. His sense of himself as a man may change because of an operation he's had or hormonal changes his treatment may have caused. He may be in too much pain to even consider sex and need every ounce of energy just to stay alive.

On the flip side of that, your husband may require more intimacy, physical contact, and sex to feel physically present, alive, and viable, no matter what his physical condition may be. He may no longer be able to have intercourse but will desire gratification in other ways. Either way, this may create changes or more problems and stresses for you.

If your husband no longer wants sex, you might feel relieved. But for Cathy and Susan, that was not the case. Craig and Sam were still able to have sex but never wanted it. Tom wasn't able, but he enjoyed special attention from Tina, and just giving that attention was sufficient for her. Fran and Frank had an Understanding, and for Jean and Joe and Mary and Mark, it was a non-issue, as they all seemed to be in accord.

But among that group of women, and not necessarily where you'd expect it, some of them had affairs. In each case, this happened after the illness had continued for several years. Although some of this was simply about sex and diversion, most was to compensate for the lack of physical touch, intimacy, and special attention toward the wives that they sorely missed. In some cases, when the husband's needs were more than the wife could handle, whether because of her low energy or because of his physical condition, *professional* assistance was brought in.

Staying Awake
When Trauma Becomes Normal

One of the perils of the long dying/decline process is that trauma is so frequent that it becomes our norm. We have a tendency to forget what "normal" really can be. I am reminded of this when I hear of friends who are about to have surgery, such as a hernia operation or a heart catheterization. Since this isn't their norm, they are concerned for weeks, and their entire family gathers around. Great concern is expressed, and a whole cluster of activity bursts into motion. It is a really big deal. And it is. Yet I sit back and think, "Gee, in one month, in addition to twelve dialysis sessions, my husband had two exploratory procedures on his artificial vein, a hernia repaired, and a permanent filter to trap blood clots placed in his aorta." And it was all done without much fanfare—which is a shame. Not that we want the illness to be a big deal, but sometimes so much goes on that it is easy to become numb.

There are ways to avoid that and stay awake during times like this. One very simple way is to seek out and to listen to stories from people who are having what I call "normal" lives. It is so easy for this "sick life" to become normal that we forget what it is like "out there." I used to ask my friends to tell me about the nice things they were doing, the trips they were taking, and the adventures they were having. Unfortunately, my friends were a bit reluctant to share some of this, as they thought it might make me feel bad. So I encouraged them and vicariously enjoyed what's out there. One of the wives who had her friends share their experiences received an e-mail from one saying, "I am glad you vicariously shared my nice normal day, and that shows a big heart, too."

Give yourself the luxury of watching fun TV or movies, even if you fall asleep in the middle of them. At least the thoughts you have as you drift off to sleep may be happy ones.

"Sometimes a Cigar Is Just a Cigar"

As we pass through the difficult times of our husbands' dying process, we may look for a bigger meaning to it all. Why me? Why him? What's it all about? Am I being punished? Am I being given a gift? Am I being tested? Am I paying off karma? Am I earning dharma, whatever that is?

You may or may not wish to pursue those questions. "Sometimes a cigar is just a cigar," as Freud is said to have remarked. The stress of pushing yourself to find an answer isn't one you need. I don't recommend searching for an answer. Who's to say what is the right answer, if one even exists? That being said, probably at some point you'll search anyway. If you decide to do that, a healthy approach is to review your behavior before the illness and compare it to what it is now. Do you like it better now? If it has changed for the better, recognize that so you can continue this behavior in the future. Some women find they become much more self-reliant and are proud of that. If you don't like your behavior, spending some time with Chapter 4, which introduced the concept of Understandings, will give you what you need to start changing.

Mary was extremely pleased to find that she not only had a right to but was able to communicate and take stands on issues of importance to her. Cathy, on the other hand, did not like her harsh behavior and overreactions to people, so she knew she had work to do in that area.

Health Lessons I Learned from My Husband

If a "gift" lies in this situation, it could be the chance to see what illness can do to a person and to a family. A common complaint wives have is that their husbands either could have completely prevented their diseases or done things to keep symptoms from getting worse. Most of us spend considerable time and energy talking to ourselves about this. Although a few may have angrily pointed out to their husbands that they caused their own diseases, certainly at some point all of us let our husbands know what they should be doing about it. You may have wondered why your husband doesn't see this when it is so clear to you. And it really is clear and right in front of you.

I suggest taking a good look at this clear picture, because it applies to you. I surely don't want to go through what my husband did. Do you want to go through what your husband is or was going through? The one thing we certainly are in charge of in this world is ourselves. And we can take care of ourselves. That choice is ours.

chapter 9

50 Do's and Don'ts

Knowing full well that the last thing you have a lot of is extra time, I include the most important ideas from the entire book in this chapter for a quick glance. Even though the ideas are numbered, this list is presented in no particular order. These ideas represent the highlights from my medical psychotherapy practice, my personal journey, and the wisdom of the six other women in this book who took a similar journey.

Once a day, or once every few days, jump in anywhere. Pick just one idea as a reminder to yourself. Or look at several. Think of a number, and go to that item. Go forward or backward in the list. Start at the end or the middle. See which ideas catch your attention. The ideas that catch your attention probably are the reminders you need the most on that particular day.

Although the majority of these concepts are self-focused, using them will help create the possibility that you and your husband can make it through these challenges, including the death itself, emotionally whole and with compassion for yourself and for each other. That is the major goal toward which everything in this book is directed.

1. Don't let your husband, or anyone, take advantage of you or be abusive to you in any way. Illness is never an excuse for brutality, whether verbal or physical.

2. Don't be afraid to ask for help wherever or however you feel you need it. If you can afford hired help, insist on it. If you can't, then ask friends, family, and agencies for help.

3. Don't feel guilty that you still have a life and still can have fun. Life may not always seem fair, but that doesn't mean life is wrong.

4. Don't enable or be codependent. It doesn't become you, and it harms both you and your husband.

5. Don't procrastinate on anything that's good for you. You may think that when you get the energy you'll do something, but the energy doesn't come until you *start* doing something.

6. Don't isolate yourself for long periods of time. It is okay for a little while to stop the drain and to regenerate, but you also need to connect with people.

7. Don't take on roles and jobs just because somebody thinks you should. You are the boss of yourself.

8. Don't worry about trying to change other people's opinions. You don't have to make them wrong for you to be right. And it is fine to agree to disagree.

9. Do take advantage of the time you have with your husband. Do as much together as you can now, so you have fewer regrets and more nice things to remember.

10. Do use the communication and antistress tools from this book. You can create a better quality of life for both of you. You don't have to do this the hard way.

11. Do recognize that he's the one dying, not you. If the situation were reversed, what would he do?

12. Do know that his journey and your journey are not one and the same. You've got different things for which to prepare, so don't get lost on his path.

13. Do realize that even if you sacrifice yourself completely, it won't stop him from dying. The result would just be two dead people instead of one.

14. Do speak up for yourself, using your communication tools, and take a hard line on safety issues. Although you have no control over many things, you still do over some aspects.

15. Do look at the humor in your mutual imperfection and try to laugh rather than to criticize. This applies to you as well as to your husband.

16. Do learn relaxation methods, such as deep breathing, hypnosis, imagery, or meditation. Not only will they help you, but your husband may see you using them and want to try them, too.

17. Don't be embarrassed about your husband's illness. It has nothing to do with your character or how good a wife you are.

18. Do give your husband a way to communicate, so you don't have to run all the time—a whistle, a bell, an air horn, a call button, an emergency button, a walkie-talkie, or a cell phone. Frustration and stress for both of you will drop, while safety will increase.

19. Do have fun where and how you can with your husband. The good endorphins will help you both.

20. Do have fun anyway, even if he can't participate. You'll both benefit.

21. Do stay active and social. If you're invited to something as a

couple and you know your husband won't be well enough to attend, ask if your host minds if you come alone.

22. Do take care of your health. What have you got to lose?

23. Do find a way to get sleep, regardless of whether or not your husband can. Trying to stay awake whenever he is awake may cause sleep deprivation for you and make you less able to take care of him.

24. Do keep connections with your friends. These will be your lifeline.

25. Do spend time with people who make you feel better, and don't spend time with people who make you feel "less than" or worse. Time is precious, so choose wisely.

26. Do eat well. Besides giving you energy, healthy food will give you the nutrients to create natural stress inhibitors and antidepressants.

27. Do physical activity regularly. It will give you more energy and help your body produce natural antidepressants.

28. Do keep your spiritual connection. Whatever it may be, it can give you strength and calmness.

29. Do pay attention so that when traumas become part of normalcy, you'll awaken and realize you need to do something about this. Expose yourself to healthy and happy things, whether in the lives of friends or on TV.

30. Do take breaks and trips and visit friends, for your well-being. Your husband might even like a break from you!

31. Do take a real respite for yourself. Let people know not to contact you during that time, or you won't get the break you need.

32. Do update health and financial planning for your husband and for yourself. Sometimes what we think we created isn't what we did or doesn't fit our current situation.

33. Do offer care alternatives for your husband during times you plan to be gone. This way you'll feel comfortable in having done what you could for his care, and he may choose what to do with it.

34. Do get support. Mother Teresa's position has already been filled.

35. Do as much funeral planning ahead of time as possible. Not only is it practical, but it can be a beautiful and intimate shared experience with your husband.

36. Do make things as easy as possible when you can. Products like Depends were created for a reason.

37. Do anger work when needed, or even when you're not sure, so it doesn't catch up with you. Anger robs your energy and may make you sick.

38. Do create a change of pace for yourself one day or night a week. As they say, even God rested on the seventh day.

39. Do protect yourself physically. Don't try to catch your husband if he's falling. If he goes down, you'll go down, too. Life will be easier if you aren't dealing with a broken arm or hip on top of doing everything else.

40. Do get away from your husband, even permanently, if it comes to a choice between him and you. You *do* have a choice.

41. Do ask lots of questions. Find somebody you trust, and get answers or opinions from that person. You don't have to figure out everything yourself.

42. Do have rote responses ready, such as "He's doing as well as can be expected. Thanks for asking." Remove some overload by not having to think on your feet.

43. Do consider warning others of your husband's appearance or medically related behavior problems so they aren't

shocked when they see him. Neither you nor your husband needs to see strong negative reactions.

44. Do get help for your depression and grief, remembering that these will occur *before* death arrives. Feelings are neither good nor bad, they just are...but you can do something about them.

45. Do consider journaling or letter writing to release uncomfortable thoughts and feelings. No sense carrying extra baggage.

46. Do create Understandings, as they are what will make life work. Make them with yourself, too, as this act will give your needs the important attention they deserve.

47. Do turn a deaf ear. People will say a lot of stupid and annoying things to you over the years, and it is better if you can let those things just float on by.

48. Do realize you won't be perfect. You weren't before, so why would that change now?

49. Do get help for yourself if you sense you are going to be verbally or physically abusive to your husband. It happens, so don't let it.

50. Do make sure that what you say improves upon the silence. Your life will be nicer because of it.

chapter *10*

Decisions, Transitions, and Discoveries

WITH ALL THE SYSTEM FAILURES my husband endured, he finally reached the point where he'd had enough. Although most people don't think of dialysis as life support, it is. To that end, my husband decided to stop dialysis. He knew that once he did, he would only have five to ten days to live.

It was a very difficult and very brave decision on his part, which he pondered constantly and gravely for more than four months. Several times he told me he would go off dialysis by a certain time, and I'd begin preparing for that, canceling all previous plans. Then he'd change his mind, and I'd prepare for return to our "normalcy." Then he'd say he wasn't going off dialysis at all. Then he'd pick another time to stop. Then he'd change his mind again. And again and again and again and again. Sometimes he wanted to tell people, and then other times he wanted to keep it secret. His final decision was to keep it secret, except for the immediate family. That made it even more difficult to put on a happy face for the world.

Finally, we had to create an Understanding about his deliberations, because his understandable vacillation created too much of a roller-coaster ride for me. Although I knew it was his decision and I would support him no matter what he decided, he changed his mind so many times that I believed he would stay on dialysis permanently. So I took myself off the roller coaster. The Understanding was that rather than continue to drag me through the process, he would let me know when he had decided. When he finally made his decision, I asked if there was anything he wanted me to do. His response was, "Believe me." I did.

He was fine for three days, which we expected, because he had gone that long without dialysis during hurricanes. On the fourth day, hospice delivered a hospital bed, a wheelchair, a walker, and various medical supplies. Because we knew this was the end, the rest of life stopped while we prepared for his transition.

Because we liked to spend the time before dinner sitting on our porch talking and watching the waterfowl land on the lake, I wheeled my husband out one Monday evening to enjoy the beautiful Florida weather. It was a lovely and special occasion that day. Of course, it was bittersweet knowing it might be the last time we were able to share this special time of our day. When he was ready to go in, he wanted to walk rather than be taken in by wheelchair. He actually *asked* for the walker—the first time he ever agreed to use one. In hindsight, I think he knew it would be the last time he'd have the chance to walk, and he didn't want to let that slip by. A proud Marine, he wanted to appear strong to the end. The determination and grit that got him through all the years of illness came into play again. He walked to his bed—and never got out of it again.

Although he hadn't asked me to do it, I had promised him many months earlier that I would protect him until the end. I didn't allow anyone to do anything to him, or about him, that I knew he wouldn't want. At this point he seemed a bit agitated, which the hospice doctor said was normal. Along with giving him medications to keep him comfortable, I began using calming and happy imagery with him. He enjoyed that. I helped him imagine being with all the dogs he had loved. This calmed and comforted him, and we progressed through other images based on his needs and thoughts at the time. He believed in heaven and had received last rites, but I still sensed some emotional distress. He seemed concerned about reaching some place with "cleansing water." He was too heavily medicated or too far gone to explain that, but I thought it might have been something he felt was a required step to get into heaven. I took him through a variety of images based on the little he told me, and this seemed to calm him, make him smile, and even chuckle on occasion.

By the next day, he had stopped speaking. Even though he had done many things that had annoyed the hell out of me during our life together, and he had done certain other things involving others in his life that he regretted, it struck me that this all was weighing very heavily on him. I felt that in the entire scheme of things, none of it was that important. Certainly, if he believed in hell, none of what he had done seemed to warrant damnation. But maybe he was worried about that. It occurred to me that that was why he had the concern about the "cleansing water." Regardless of whether I was correct or not, I felt it wouldn't hurt to try to do something about it. So each time I cleared his medicine lines with saline, I told him I was putting in "cleansing water." Although he was unresponsive, I thought he could still hear me, as hospice said hearing is the last sense to go. Of course I had already repeatedly told him I loved him, but I also began telling him he was a good man and that he deserved to go to heaven. I forgave him for anything he may have done and asked him to forgive me for anything I had done to him. The rest of the moments while he slipped further and further away, I cleansed his face, stroked him, and spoke soothingly to him.

Although his transition process left him motionless for most of the day, gradually, and with muscles quivering from the strain, he managed to move. He raised the arm I was touching until his hand touched his heart—and then he was gone. He had signaled his final good-bye. It was the end of the fifth day.

✿

A question the women I interviewed asked me several times is, "Do you think you'll feel differently about all this after your husband dies?" In response I would always say, "I don't think so, but we'll have to see." In our frank conversations, we noted that it was not uncommon for a woman, once her husband died, to elevate him to sainthood. No matter what he had done, no matter what she had gone through with him—now that he had departed, he was a saint. The grandmother in *The Sopranos* delivers a stunning portrayal of that. Her husband had been terrible in countless ways, including being a murderer, but repeatedly and emphatically she'd say, "Your father—he was a saint!"

The answer to the interviewees' question is "no." No, I haven't elevated my husband to sainthood. And, no, I don't feel different about anything in this book now that he's gone. Actually, I feel even more strongly about everything I wrote and every idea I share. I discovered dramatically and unequivocally that the methods I created and teach not only work but can dramatically improve the time you and your husband have left. For me, the result was that at the time of my husband's death, I had absolutely no regrets, and I wouldn't have done a single thing differently— and I still feel that way. Because of the process of creating Understandings, I was able to give him every suggestion I thought would help. I don't have to look back and think, "I wish I had said X to him," or "I wish I had shared Y and Z." All the things I wanted to say were said. Additionally, we didn't have to fight over them; he could decide whether or not to use them, and I could decide what I would do based on his decision. And I didn't have to be afraid to offer a suggestion, because I had a compassionate format within which to present it. Anything I wanted to say or anything he wanted to say was put on the table for discussion, and an Understanding was formulated. If he didn't choose to follow my suggestions, at least I knew I had suggested everything I could think of. I made my points, but by doing it through the process of creating Understandings, the household was more harmonious and far more pleasant. And because we created Understandings, we kept our integrity in regard and in response to his health care and his medical conditions. Finally, because I used the four-category sorting process described in Chapter 2, I don't regret anything I said.

Yet I discovered one more idea at the end that I'll share with you now. Although the Understandings created peace in the house and an exceedingly better life than would have been imaginable without them, a few didn't always create peace in my heart. The car driving Understanding is a good example, as my husband was still driving within two weeks of his passing. However, in finally knowing the time frame for his departure, an opportunity was created for me. It was as if a switch was flipped when I sensed his distress about the heaven issue. I saw an opportunity to perform some final acts of kindness, compassion, and love—ones that were far beyond those I normally would have considered. With everything now in a different perspective, and in acting to quell my sense of his distress, the amazing result was that all the anger and all the annoyance that I had been storing was gone. Not gone because he died. Not gone now because I was empty. Gone because the emotions had been replaced with peace, thanks to my final words and actions.

So how does this apply to you? You may not know the exact time frame for when your husband will pass. Yet, you have another way to create this opportunity. I would suggest that every night while your husband is asleep, no matter how angry you are at him or how rotten he has been, you whisper the things to him you'd say if you knew it were his last day. You may be so annoyed with him that you want to be sure he doesn't really hear the nice things, so you may go to another room or go outside, if that's what you need to do to be able to say them. And, yes, he'll awaken the next morning and annoy the hell out of you, make demands, and do all the unacceptable behaviors again and again. And that's all right, because there *will* be one morning when he doesn't awaken. It may make no difference for him that you say those things, but it will make a difference for *you*. If you do this, you'll be able to have peace in your heart. It *does* "improve upon the silence."

Resources

Resource sections at the back of books have an inherent drawback. The information included often is, or quickly becomes, out of date. It is also not local. For the most up-to-date information, the first resource about your husband's disease or terminal condition and what you should do about it is his physician or primary caregiver (and their medical staff). This person should be able to supply their knowledge along with pamphlets and other materials detailing the condition, including phone numbers, addresses, and websites for local and national assistance regarding every aspect of care and support.

Like it or not, the computer probably is going to be your greatest resource for gathering comprehensive information. Accessing volumes of information is much easier than in years past and will constantly lead you to the most current information. Because of this, I decided that rather than giving you a fish, I would teach you to fish. Rather than listing in this Resource section every place to gain access to information on every possible illness, support group, or agency related thereto, I'll teach you how to do computer searches and suggest topics for which you may want to search. These computer searches may have been difficult and frustrating for you, or just annoying on a good day. But they are well worth the effort, and understanding how to perform them will make this work for you.

Before I begin teaching the computer-research process, let me provide you with some noncomputer ways to find information.

In a Crisis

9-1-1—Probably everyone knows that 9-1-1 is the easiest and most direct resource in a medical or police emergency. But some areas are not served by 9-1-1. If you live in one of those areas, as I did, be sure you have the phone numbers for your police, ambulance, fire/rescue, hospital, and doctors posted near several phones in your house.

On-Star—If your car is equipped with this service or you have it on your cell phone, it may be able to connect you to a variety of emergency services and information sources at the time of a crisis.

2-1-1—The Federal Communications Commission (FCC) selected the telephone number 2-1-1 for easy access to community human service information. Forty-six states now have call centers answering 2-1-1 calls. These centers provide information about where to get help in local communities. As mentioned in Chapter 5, if you are starting to act abusively toward your husband, you need to get help right away. 2-1-1, linked to the United Way, is a number to call to find a resource for any crisis intervention. Additionally, 2-1-1 provides free and confidential information on food, housing, health care, counseling, disability, senior care, addictions, and much more. It is available 24/7.

Get Noncrisis Information Without the Computer

Obviously, you can look in the phone book to access numbers and addresses for local resources, but that may require a lot of walking with your fingers. An oft-forgotten source of information is your local newspaper, in which you may find listings for community support meetings, such as those for caregivers or various medical conditions, or announcements for special conferences currently taking place in your community. Local television and radio stations typically have public service commitments and may gladly direct you to the information you need. Religious institutions, public libraries, city halls, and hospitals either provide, post notices about, or run support or information groups, as do local mental-health associations and colleges. These are places you may visit in person or simply call.

How to Do Computer Searches

This process does take time, but you'll find it well worth the effort once you learn a few simple concepts. When I search, I usually stumble upon additional important information or resources I never knew existed. So the seemingly dead ends or long lists I encounter in this process are usually rich with information. Be patient. If you're really having trouble, ask someone under the age of twelve for help—they will find the information on your computer in a flash!

What do you want to know? In the "search" box (a rectangular box that usually says "search" just after it) on your Internet home page, type in what you want to know, being as specific as possible. The search program (called a search engine) uses the main words you entered to find things for you. You don't have to form a sentence, use capital letters, or even spell perfectly. But don't worry if you're used to writing whole sentences, because the computer will ignore the unimportant words. After you type in your words or sentence, press the "Enter" key.

For example, if you want to find caregiver support groups in Omaha, Nebraska, all you have to type is "caregiver support groups Omaha Nebraska." If you want to find caregiver support groups for muscular dystrophy in Omaha, Nebraska, just add "muscular dystrophy" to what you type, either at the beginning or the end. If you don't have money, need legal services, and live in Oshkosh, Wisconsin, type "legal services no money Oshkosh Wisconsin" and hit the "Enter" key.

What happens next is that your computer displays a list. You'll notice that the first line of each item usually is underlined or in bold print. That's because a website address is hidden (embedded) in it. It is good to remember this, because as you look through material at any site, you'll run into these underlined or bolded phrases or words. This almost always means you may click on those words and automatically be taken to more specific information. The good thing is that you don't have to bother with the Internet address, those "http://" and "www" things that I'll briefly explain later.

You'll also notice along the bottom of the screen that numbers in little boxes indicate the presence of many more pages. The search engine usually sorts the list it gives you by relevance and shows the most relevant items first. It is usually a waste of time to go beyond the second or third page of results. Taking the legal services in Oshkosh, Wisconsin, as an example, I found forty-seven pages, including how a credit card was charged illegally at a hotel and legal notices about a sub shop.

Notice also that a listing at the top or bottom of the page may be in a colored block. Usually this means that the website owner has paid to have its listing in a prominent place on the page.

Now that you're at the list, skim the subject lines to see if one looks like what you want. If one does, click on that underlined or bolded wording to be taken directly to a page of information on that topic. As you'll see below, it might be a lot of information, and I'll teach you how to move through that. If you're in the wrong area, use the "back" arrow on your screen to return to the previous page. But if it looks like you're in the right topic area, it is time to move around the page a bit to find more.

Website Terms

At the top of the page, just below the main title, along the left side, or sometimes at the bottom, you'll see a list of items. If you click on any of the words, it usually will take you to a place that explains something. Below are the typical words you'll see, along with an explanation of each.

About Us — This section offers general information about what an organization or company does. The specifics are listed elsewhere. It may give you names of the people who are in charge of that organization, but many sites do not provide names.

Contact Us — Although a company or organization sometimes puts its address and phone number on the top or bottom of the opening page, often it does not. To find out phone and fax numbers or the mailing addresses, look here. What you may find is a form to fill out, on your computer, that will send an e-mail directly to the company without your having to open your e-mail program. What you may find from larger companies that sell products, such as wheelchairs, for example, is that when you go to "Contact Us," you will see a list of departments to choose from—do you want sales, repair, technical support, etc?—so you must take one further step to get to the right place. Often, companies that sell a product don't provide representatives to speak directly to you and require that you fill out an e-mail form if you seek information. But that usually is not the case for any organization or group that deals with a specific disease, caregiving services, or support groups.

Live Chat—The word "chat" is used pretty loosely here, because it is not done on the phone. Instead, you'll type a question into a little screen or window that is displayed on your computer, and the other person will type an answer into the screen on their computer, which you'll soon see on your little screen. You continue in this manner as long as needed.

Programs and Services or Products—In the case of organizations, when you click on this category, another list of words will drop down under the one you just clicked on. It is actually called a "drop-down list." This will give you more options from which to choose. Just click on the one that interests you, and you'll end up at a page with that information. If you didn't find what you want, use the "Back" arrow and try again. In the case of a company that sells products—let's say wheelchairs again—a drop-down list might include motorized, sports, ultralight, and other terms that describe the various types of wheelchairs it sells.

Mission—Most organizations and some companies tell you their purpose. It is often helpful to read this. For instance, you may go to a site about caregivers, but when you read the posted mission statement, you learn the company's purpose is help find employment for people who want to be caregivers. This likely isn't what you were looking for.

Search—Just like the area on your Internet browser's home page, you will type in the information you're trying to find. The difference is that this usually keeps the search within the site you're viewing rather than opening it to the entire World Wide Web. Let's say you came to a page for muscular dystrophy caregiver support groups for California and you live in San Diego. You would type "San Diego" into that search box.

Information—This likely provides specific details about the organization or company and what it does or will tell you where to find that information. It usually is not going to provide a place for you to ask your specific question to get the information you want.

F.A.Q.—This stands for "Frequently Asked Questions." Because companies and organizations often receive the same questions over and over and over again, they list those questions along with answers to them. Sometimes these questions are printed in bold type or underlined. As mentioned before, that means you may click on them to get to the answers.

Site Map—Sometimes this is a fast resource, as it provides a simple list of the main items on a website. Simply find your item and click on it to be taken directly to that topic.

Get Help or Help—Often you won't see this. Instead, use "Contact Us." When this option is offered, it may take you to F.A.Q. (see the definition above). Generally, "Help" isn't very helpful, and you'll need to use "Contact Us" to get the information you need for your particular situation.

These are the common terms, although you'll find more along the top and sides of Web pages. At this point, most should be self-explanatory.

"http://," "WWW," "URL," and all those symbols—If you have the Internet address for an organization or company, you have its "URL," or Universal Resource Locator. That's the address you enter near the very top of your screen. Now if someone offers to give you a URL, you'll know what the person means. It often begins with "http," which stands for "hyper text protocol"—and which you may now forget, because you'll never need to know that. If the URL begins with "www," you probably already know that means "World Wide Web." I am mentioning these because usually you don't need to use them to enter an Internet address. As an example, even though the correct URL for Al-Anon is "http://www.al-anon .alateen.org," all I need to enter to go directly to the site is "al-anon .com." The computer makes corrections and fills in all the extra letters, making it easier for us. You'll find that unlike sites for companies whose URLs end in ".com" (for "commercial"), many of the places you will go to end in ".org" (for organization) or ".edu" (an educational institution).

"Pop-Ups"—Hopefully you have pop-ups, those little ads and notices that just appear on your screen from out of nowhere, blocked (if you don't know how to check this setting on your computer, ask someone to show you how to do so). The downside of this is that when you click on some of those underlined or bolded items, you'll see a notice that the pop-up is blocked. This simply means that you need to temporarily remove the block for this information to appear. This shouldn't happen very often in the type of searches you'll be doing regarding your husband's illness. Never "allow" the pop-up if you are afraid the source might not be legitimate.

Facebook and Twitter—Organizations usually have a Facebook or Twitter page. Although these are quite popular, I recommend using regular Internet searches instead, as Facebook and Twitter were designed to be social networks. Because the general public may add information and comments to these pages, often it is difficult to wade through everything to find the information you need. But if you like using Facebook or Twitter, it might be an additional alternative.

What Can or Should I Search For?

As a woman whose husband is dying, certain topics may be of particular interest to you. Below are suggested ideas for your searches. These are issues that may or may not have come into your mind before, but now they certainly will.

Once you've found the information you want, I suggest doing two things right away. The first is adding the page to your favorites, which some call "bookmarking." Near the top of your screen you may see the words "Bookmarks" or "Favorites." Click on the word and you should see wording such as "Add to Favorites" or "Bookmark Page." If you click on the option, a little window will open asking permission to do so. Click on "Add" or "Yes." This way, when you decide you want to see it again, you won't have to start from scratch, and you can simply click on your "Favorites" or "Bookmarks" icon near the top of the screen. Surprisingly, you can enter a search word one day and produce a different list of items than the same search word would produce on another day. So don't count on being able to find it easily with the same search words.

The second thing is printing out any information you want to remember. It is much faster than trying to search for it again. There are several ways to do that. Some of your Web pages have a printer icon just above the page content, which you'll click on to print. Others have the word "print" and/or an icon of a printer at the top of the content. It is usually not easy to find, but once you've found one, you'll know what to look for in the future.

Your Mental and Emotional Health

For some of the topics I have included the contact data for the national organization, but you should seek contact information locally as well. I have also included some topics you may explore to obtain information you didn't know was available, along with a few e-mail and postal (also known as snail-mail) addresses. I've listed Mental Health America first because like this book, the organization's main focus is promoting mental and emotional health for you and your husband.

Mental Health America
2000 N. Beauregard St., 6th Fl.
Alexandria VA 22311
(800) 969-6642   (703) 684-7722
Fax: (703) 684-5968
www.nmha.org

You can look for a local branch of Mental Health America in your county: Three hundred are available nationwide. Note that due to a name change to the national organization in 2006, many of the local affiliates still go by part of the national organization's previous name, "Mental Health Association." Mental Health America affiliates bring together mental-health consumers, parents, advocates, and service providers for collaboration and action. The national association provides training and technical assistance to these affiliates on such issues as managed care, mental health–parity advocacy, anxiety-disorders and depression education, and children's mental-health issues. The national office offers local and state affiliates vital assistance in board development, fund-raising plans, and program implementation.

"Who Is a Caregiver?"

If you are looking for information to help you care for your husband, remember that the term "caregiver" has several meanings. The person who is in charge of your medical care, your physician, is now commonly referred to as your "primary caregiver." So "caregiver" may mean "doctor." Some people are paid to take care of sick people, and they also are called caregivers. Then there are those people who aren't paid for the task, and they (except not always in the case of a wife) are also called caregivers. So it is important to word your search questions specifically and be ready to look quite carefully at the search results list.

Caregiving for Husband or Partner
Example: *Caregiver Challenges: Caregiving for a Husband or Partner Who Is or Has Been Controlling or Hurtful*

www.dhs.wisconsin.gov/publications/P2/p20224a.pdf
This document offers advice for people who are caregivers for people who are controlling or abusive.

Caregiver Support Groups
Example: National Family Caregiver Support
www.agingcarefl.org/caregiver/NationalSupport
Sponsored by the National Family Caregiver Support Program (NFCSP) and funded by the federal Older Americans Act, Title III E, this organization helps people of any age who serve as unpaid caregivers for people ages sixty and older. The goal of this program is to relieve the emotional, physical, and financial hardships of providing continual care.

Codependence and Codependency Support
These topics need to be searched locally.

Al-Anon
Al-Anon World Service Office
1600 Corporate Landing Pkwy.
Virginia Beach VA 23454
www.al-anon.alateen.org

Disease-Specific Support Groups
Example: www.kidney.org/site/503/support_group.cfm?ch=503

Exercise — To Relieve Stress
Example: Mayo Clinic — www.mayoclinic.com/health/exercise
-and-stress/SR00036

Meditation — To Relieve Stress
Example: e-How — www.ehow.com/how_2226500_use-meditation
-relieve-anxiety.html

Meditation and Yoga Instruction
Example: www.kripalu.org

Self-hypnosis — To Relieve Stress
Example: http://stress.about.com/od/lowstresslifestyle/ht/Howto
selfhyp.htm

Therapists — For Caregivers or Codependents
Examples: www.caring.com/blogs/caring-currents/therapy-for
-caregivers
www.ncbi.nlm.nih.gov/pmc/articles/PMC2424274
This topic needs to be searched locally.

Yoga — To Relieve Stress
Example: Mayo Clinic — www.mayoclinic.com/health/yoga
/CM00004

Assistance with Giving Care

Examples: Caregiver.com — http://caregiver.com
Caregiver Media Group is a leading provider of information, support, and guidance for family and professional caregivers.
Medicare — http://www.medicare.gov/caregivers
Medicare provides a very comprehensive list of information about caregiver support.

Hospice
Example: http://hospicenet.org
This website provides information for patients and families facing life-threatening illnesses.

Housekeepers
This topic needs to be searched locally.

Professional Caregivers
Be careful when looking under "Medical Caregivers," because you will find many sites about medical marijuana, which may not be what you're looking for.
Example: National Association of Geriatric Care Managers —
www.caremanager.org/displaycommon.cfm?an=1&subarticle
nbr=46

Medical Information Regarding Your Husband's Disease

Disease- or Condition-Specific Nonprofit Organizations

Examples: American Diabetes Association — www.diabetes.org
United Ostomy Associations of America — www.ostomy.org
Because organizations dedicated to a specific disease have already researched and organized their material and present it in one place, it may save time to start with such a site. If you start with the name of the disease alone, the search engine will present too much information in too many different subject areas.

Medical Information Sites

Not everything is accurate. Stay with sites from major hospitals and medical schools.
Examples: Harvard — www.health.harvard.edu
Mayo Clinic — www.mayoclinic.com/health/medical/HomePage
Cleveland Clinic — www.cchs.net/hinfo

Legal and Financial Information

Estate Lawyers

Contact your state bar association.

Insurance and Financial Rights

Continue with your state bar association or legal aid.

Low-Income Legal Aid

Example for Oregon: www.osbar.org/public/ris/LowCostLegal Help/LegalAid.html

Wives' Legal Rights

Contact your state bar association.
Example for Illinois: www.illinoislawyerfinder.com/legalinfo

Government Agencies

Medicare
www.medicare.gov/caregivers

U.S. Department of Health and Human Services (HHS)
200 Independence Ave. SW
Washington DC 20201
www.hhs.gov
This organization is the U.S. government's principal agency for protecting the health of all Americans and providing essential human services, especially for those who are least able to help themselves.

National Association of Area Agencies on Aging
1730 Rhode Island Ave. NW, Ste. 1200
Washington DC 20036
(202) 872-0888
Fax: (202) 872-0057
http://n4a.org
This organization's primary mission is to build the capacity of its members to help older persons and persons with disabilities live with dignity and choices in their homes and communities for as long as possible.

Department of Elder Affairs
This agency is under HHS. Check by state for its Consumer Resource Guide (I highly recommend getting this).
Example: Florida Department of Elder Affairs
4040 Esplanade Way
Tallahassee FL 32399-7000
(850) 414-2000   TDD: (850) 414-2001
Fax: (850) 414-2004
http://elderaffairs.state.fl.us
The primary state agency administering human services programs to benefit Florida's elders.

General Information
Household Repairs
Example: *How to Be a Handywoman: A Girl's Guide to Home Repairs*

www.googobits.com/articles/2059-how-to-be-a-handywoman-a
-girl-s-guide-to-home-repairs.html

Household First-Aid
Examples:
First-aid kits: http://firstaid.webmd.com/first-aid-kits-treatment
How to give a shot: www.drugs.com/cg/how-to-give-an-intra
muscular-injection.html
How to do CPR: http://depts.washington.edu/learncpr/quickcpr
.html
Getting blood out of a carpet: www.ehow.com/how_5061000
_blood-stains-out-carpet.html

Driving Ability
Example: www.driveable.com

Dialysis at Sea
www.dialysisatsea.com

Local Radio and Television Stations

Check for community outreach, family, relationship, religion, and
other departments.

Books

American Medical Association and Angela Perry, eds. *American
Medical Association Guide to Home Caregiving.* Hoboken, NJ: John
Wiley & Sons, Inc., 2001.

Canfield, Jack, Mark Victor Hansen, and LeAnn Thieman. *Chicken
Soup for the Caregiver's Soul: Stories to Inspire Caregivers in the Home,
Community and the World.* Deerfield Beach, FL: Health Communi-
cations, Inc., 2004.

Sheehy, Gail. *Passages in Caregiving: Turning Chaos into Confidence.*
New York: William Morrow, 2010.

Melody Beattie's many books on codependency

Index